SHAPE YOUR SELF

SHAPE YOUR SELF

My 6-Step Diet and Fitness Plan to Achieve the Best Shape of Your Life

MARTINA NAVRATILOVA

RODALE

© 2006 by Martina Navratilova

Printed in the United States of America
Rodale Inc. makes every effort to use acid-free ∞, recycled paper ♻.

Interior photographs by Mitch Mandel
Interior photography art direction by Patricia Field

Book design by Christina Gaugler

Library of Congress Cataloging-in-Publication Data

Navratilova, Martina, date.
    Shape your self: my 6-step diet and fitness plan to achieve the best shape of your life / Martina Navratilova.
       p.   cm.
    Includes index.
    ISBN-13 978–1–59486–282–3 hardcover
    ISBN-10 1–59486–282–6 hardcover
    1. Health—Popular works.   2. Physical fitness—Popular works.   3. Nutrition—Popular works.
4. Weight loss—Popular works.   I. Title.
    RA776.N38   2006
    613.7—dc22   2005033103

Distributed to the trade by Holtzbrinck Publishers

      4   6   8   10   9   7   5   3   hardcover

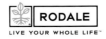

We inspire and enable people to improve their lives and the world around them

For more of our products visit **rodalestore.com** or call 800-848-4735

Throughout my life, I have experienced some of the best and the worst in human nature—in romance, in business, and even in friendships. To date, I don't know anyone who has been slam-dunked as much as I have, except for maybe a basketball. Even so, I have also had the great fortune to cross paths with some of the most amazing individuals on Earth, especially one person who is someone pretty darn special. When I wanted to dedicate this book to her, she asked me not to do that but to instead dedicate it to all those who inspire others, not just in word but in deed, because she wouldn't be my inspiration if she had not been inspired by others. She reminded me that I too had those people in my own life who told me I could when others told me I couldn't . . . people who inspired me to keep going when others told me to give up.

So I dedicate this book to people who inspire others to be the very best they can be and to our elders who live by example, inspiring in all of us important values such as honesty, integrity, fairness, and truth.

CONTENTS

ACKNOWLEDGMENTS

First and foremost, I wish to thank all my fans. It is because of you that this book was written. You kept asking me, "Martina, how do you stay so fit? Why are you in such great shape? What do you eat?" I guess I got tired of answering these questions by saying, "It's my way of life!" And so this book was born.

Next, I have a long list of other "thank-yous," so please bear with me!

Thank you to my one and only best friend for sharing a lot of stories with me, some of which are in the book, and for her infinite wisdom. Thank you for doing a lot more than that and never taking a penny or a dollar, for that matter.

Thank you, Jeremy Steindecker, my agent and a great guy who pushed me into writing this book, for your valuable input and ideas throughout the whole process.

Thank you, Maggie Greenwood-Robinson, for putting all the thoughts, ideas, stories, recipes, and exercises into an organized form and for your input.

Thank you, Lisa Austin, for your help with the exercise chapter.

Thank you, Heather Jackson and Mariska van Aalst, for giving this book all the right trimmings, including help with format, order, and information.

Thank you, Rodale Books staff, for your research, great photos, and recipe testing.

Thank you, Salton, for the Juiceman and all your great recipes (the Juiceman is a juicer that just did not quit when I tried them all out!).

Thank you, SPRI Products, for such great exercise tools. It was only after getting the idea for the "all at home" workout program that I started looking for the equipment for it and found that SPRI has it all.

Thank you, Under Armour clothing, for making Lisa and me look great in the exercise photos (if I do say so myself!).

Thank you, Linda Dozoretz, my publicist, for your friendship and all your help through the years. (Actually, it was Linda who had the idea for this book years ago, but I didn't think there was much interest at the time.)

Thank you, Warren Bosworth, who had nothing to do with this book but was always in my corner. By the way, you make great tennis racquets!

Thank you, Thor-Lo Socks. I have not worn anything else on my feet since 1981 and thus have some of the best-looking feet in the tennis world!

Thank you, Pat Cairns at Oakley, for keeping the wrinkles around my eyes to a minimum by always sending me great sunglasses.

Thank you, Pat and Corey McLernon, caretakers with a capital C.

Thank you, Annie Leibovitz, for letting me use your photo and making me look so good (again, if I do say so myself).

Thank you, Robin, for just being you.

And last but certainly not least, thank you, readers, for having enough faith in me to buy this book—or did you borrow it from a friend? Either way, you are reading it, and hopefully that means you are getting in the best shape of your life.

Martina

P.S. Please visit me at my Web site, www.martinanavratilova.com, and let me know about your progress!

BECAUSE I CAN . . . AND SO CAN YOU

The ball doesn't know how old I am.

There I was, running sprints on the track at a local high school to improve my speed on the tennis court. Nearby, a group of 14-year-old boys watched me go through drill after drill. One of the boys spoke up, "Whose mom is that? She's really cool."

Well, I don't know how "cool" I looked, and I'm not a mom, except to 15 purebreds and mutts (dogs, of course!). But I do know that I can outrun many women who are half my age, still play tennis competitively, and do all the other sports I love: basketball, hockey, and skiing, to name a few. I'm not ashamed to admit it: I do feel young.

As I approach that milestone of 50, I've been asked hundreds of times, "Why can you still move the way you do? How do you stay in such good shape? What's your secret?"

My "secret" has been a combination of things. I follow a healthy, delicious diet. I pay attention when little aches and pains pop up, and I take care of them. I work out and play lots of different sports. I take time off from my workouts. Along with all that, there's hard work, a little common sense, and some genetic luck thrown in for good measure. My formula, lifestyle, philosophy, or whatever else you want to call it has evolved from more than 30 years of trial and error, fortunately more successful trial than error. I've worked with nutritionists, trainers, coaches, doctors, osteopaths, chiropractors, homeopaths, and kinesiologists. You name it, I have probably tried it! I've taken the best of what they've taught me and made it work for me. Through my many years of experimentation and application, I've found what I believe is the best way to shape your self, inside and out.

Does this involve a strict diet of nothing but rabbit food? No.

Hours and hours of working out? Again, no.

How about quick fixes for breaking bad habits? Fugeddaboudit!

What it does involve is a series of small, gradual changes—put into a step-by-step strategy—that I know you can do without ever feeling deprived or getting frustrated. When followed, these strategies will give you more energy, a body that works—and looks—a lot better, fitness you can see and feel, and an inner shift that will make good health a permanent part of your life. This is neither a fad nor an overnight program. It's a way of life—one that helps you achieve balance in your life, with the physical, mental, and emotional all working in harmony. It's how I've achieved the shape of my life.

Let me ask you some questions to start you thinking: Does it matter to you if you're overweight? That you feel lousy, day in and day out? That you're dragging yourself around, not being able to do what you want to do? That your quality of life isn't as good as it should be? For some people, obviously, it doesn't matter.

But I believe that if you're reading this book, it *does* matter to you. One of my mantras is: If it matters, you don't mind it.

So if it matters to you to get in the shape of your life—and I hope that's your aim—then you won't mind the small lifestyle changes or tiny sacrifices it takes to get there. Hey, I don't necessarily like running those sprints or taking the time to stretch after a workout, but I know it's necessary to get better, to get in better shape, to get to the ball—so I can win that match! I like getting the most out of my body because it helps me get the most out of my life.

This book is all about victory—yours! I promise if you stay with me through every word, taking what you learn and applying what you need, you'll begin to look good and feel better, physically and mentally. You'll dig within yourself, unearth your inner strength, and achieve championship levels in every area of your life.

WHAT'S AGE GOT TO DO WITH IT?

Getting in shape really starts with this advice: Don't let age get in your way. Don't let age define your identity or govern what you can or cannot do. Look at your ability, not at your age.

As an athlete, I had to deal with age and aging very early. For most female athletes, 30 is the age at which you should be retired. Your career is over. You are past your peak, finished.

I guess I never bought into the notion that my best tennis, or my best anything, for that matter, was behind me or finished. What a depressing thought. Sure, you have to make some concessions to age, but you don't have to give in to it. Honestly, I feel that I'm a better tennis player now than I was 20 years ago, maybe just not as fast or as strong because of my age. And I'm always striving to play even better. I know I can still improve my technique, learn more about what kind of shots to hit, and work on my strategy. Through it all, I can't wait to see where I can next take my game, my body, or my life.

While you can't escape the fact that your body will slow down, your fitness, health, and energy can get better with each passing year, whether you're 25 or 55. It won't happen automatically, and it won't happen overnight. But don't panic. If you make the effort, you'll feel a difference within a week or two at the most. It just takes a deep-down desire to improve your life.

You don't feel old merely because you have lived a certain number of years. You feel old when you abandon the desire to be better than you are—and that can happen at any age. I've wanted to improve ever since I started hitting tennis balls against a cement wall as a $4\frac{1}{2}$-year-old court rat. I didn't figure out how to hit a topspin backhand until I was 26, and it's been only recently that I've developed a more versatile forehand. Now, here I am, and I think my strokes are technically better than ever. If you didn't know I was 49 years old, if you didn't know my name was Martina Navratilova, you'd say, "Hey, that's a pretty good tennis player out there!"

But beyond tennis, I'm eating smarter than ever before. I'm drinking more fresh juices, and I've added more raw foods to my diet. I've learned brand-new cardio, strength, agility, and flexibility exercises that I never knew existed, many of which I'll share with you in this book. I've gotten better at enlisting all levels of my being—mind, body, and spirit—to become a better person, someone who strives to make a positive difference in this world. Certainly, I have a long way to go, but what keeps me going is pushing the envelope and trying to find out what my limits really are. Isn't that what makes any endeavor fun, rewarding, and ultimately worth pursuing?

FOOD, FITNESS, AND ME

Two of the topics I'll be talking about a lot in this book are nutrition and exercise. Your body is a gift, and it's important to take care of it—not just for yourself but also so you can take care of others. If we treat our bodies properly by giving them healthy food and the right amount of physical activity, they will return the favor. They will pay us back in energy, vitality, a clear mind, and a clean bill of health.

I do have a system for how I eat, but it's not rigid. I love food because it gives me the energy and stamina to play tennis and other sports and keep going. But I also love the sensations of food, its flavors and textures. More than anything, I love to try new cuisines. I'm a big fan of Thai and Indian food, for example, and I love to go to new restaurants. I had no exposure to different cuisines when I was growing up in the Czech Republic (it used to be called Czechoslovakia, and I think we should have stayed one country, but at least my homeland is now easier to spell). There was one very expensive Chinese restaurant in Prague, and that was it for the whole country. The Czech cuisine is quite delicious but also pretty bland, made with very few spices. Its flavors are very subtle.

Until I came to the States, I had never tasted fresh pineapple, mango (I had never heard of a mango!), asparagus, lobster, or shrimp—even cornflakes! (As I write this, I'm in Australia in January, and the mangoes are in season. Is it possible to O.D. on them? I just might find out!) I had never seen fresh basil, never heard of coriander, and never tasted red or green curry, so I really appreciate the variety of foods and spices so easily available to us, and I look forward to every meal. Some people eat to live; some live to eat. I pretty much fall into the latter category.

To many people, though, food is the enemy. They feel guilty eating it, or they think that a bite will lead to a binge. I don't get it, really. As long as you put your eating habits in order, you can enjoy food and use it to create a healthy, energetic body. Don't ever feel deprived, even if there are some foods or drinks you can't have. Instead, think of all the foods you can eat; think of all the amazing juices and smoothies you can make.

I grew up eating traditional Czech dishes. Meals were spread out over the day, which is the way most good athletes eat. We "grazed," in other words. I've always hated being hungry because it makes me feel crabby, and I've never been able to function on an empty stomach. When you graze, you don't get hungry, and you feel more energetic.

For breakfast back then, I'd have tea and wholesome rye bread with butter and jam. At school, between the second and third classes, I'd have a snack that my mom had made—a small sandwich with salami or, on a special day, ham. I ate lunch in the school cafeteria. It began with a light, brothy soup followed by a main course of boiled beef or pork and potatoes or dumplings. Very seldom did we have chicken because it was expensive—more expensive than other meats. Then, at 4:00 p.m., I'd have another small sandwich or yogurt and maybe a homemade doughnut or slice of apple strudel (yum!).

At home, dinner started with a light soup with a few veggies or dumplings in it. The main course was boiled meat, often with a light sauce made with the broth from the meat, accompanied by rice, potatoes, or dumplings. For vegetables, choices were limited. Cauliflower, beans, peas, and spinach were staples. I ate spinach because my dad told me I'd have muscles like Popeye. The vegetables were steamed or boiled, maybe with a dab of butter on top, but always prepared in a very healthy manner. Our meals were pretty low in fat, although occasionally for dinner, we'd have little hot dogs and mashed potatoes, which I loved. In the summer, there would be a salad, usually a sliced tomato salad or some Boston lettuce with vinegar, a little water, and salt and pepper, but no oil.

Sunday lunches were special and were the big meal of the week. My mother made goose, duck, or chicken with dumplings made from potatoes or flour, served after a soup, of course. Mom would often prepare my favorite, fruit dumplings, by wrapping apricots, strawberries, or blueberries in dough and plopping them in boiling water to cook. Sometimes I'd eat 10 of them. One time for lunch at school, I devoured 27 apricot dumplings. I piled 9 on my plate, then headed back for seconds and thirds because I liked them so much. But I was skinny as a rail back then—my father called me "Stick"—as were most of the kids at my school. There were really no fat kids in my class, with the exception of two classmates who were a little chubby but not so overweight that you'd say, "Those kids could lose some weight."

It's certainly not that way now in America, where childhood obesity is a major health problem. A few years ago, I was in Washington, D.C., to lobby on behalf of the sporting goods industry to obtain government funds so the industry could continue to supply public schools with sports equipment. When funding for schools is slashed, athletic programs typically get cut first, with the arts and theater falling by the wayside next. This is a real shame because we need all of these programs so badly. It was in Washington that I first learned these shocking facts: About 30 percent of children and teenagers in this country are overweight, and 15 percent are considered obese. (It's double that for adults, with 65 percent overweight and 30 percent obese.) Poor eating habits are one reason, as is inactivity. Illinois is the only state to require daily physical education classes through high school. No wonder our kids are heavy.

Recently, I visited a high school in Pennsylvania. It was a new school in a small city. Boy, was I surprised to find out that the old school gym had been demolished the year before, and the new gym wouldn't be completed for another year. This meant that the kids could not take gym class for 2 years, except for the boys on the football team, who were transported to another school so they could work out. But the other boys and girls were out of luck. This is not a good thing, needless to say. It's really hard for kids growing up in the States, particularly in our cities, to play outside and get healthy exercise. For many children, school is the only place to get any kind of physical activity.

How different it was when I was a kid growing up! I was always active. I climbed spruce trees next to our house. I started playing tennis before my fifth birthday. I ran and bicycled around our garden and pretended it was a track. I skied and played ice hockey and soccer. I was a total jock.

Through my work with the Women's Sports Foundation, I've discovered facts about how life enhancing it is for girls to be involved in sports and physical activity. For example, girls who play sports have higher self-esteem. They are less likely to smoke, use illicit drugs, be sexually active, or suffer depression. Also, they are much less likely to be in abusive relationships. They excel in school, often being selected for honors courses and going on to college. If you're a mom or dad whose kids are athletes, I applaud you.

In the Czech Republic, women had families and jobs, and they played sports. They were accustomed to using their bodies at work and at home, building up their muscles and strength. It wasn't so much a fitness mentality about diet and exercise for health's sake, as it is in the States. It was an innate sense that sport is good and a lot of fun. I grew up seeing women performing all kinds of athletics, and my mother was no different. She loved many types of sports, including tennis. She always played volleyball in my hometown's club and played tennis at our local tennis club. She did gymnastics with her friends. She skated in the winter, and of course, she skied. She was always a full-time athlete, a full-time worker, and a full-time mother. I don't know how she did it, but she made it all work. It was through my mother's example that I first learned that sports are good for young women. It's good to compete, good to run, good to sweat, good to get dirty, good to feel tired and healthy and refreshed. From the beginning, my mother was my role model.

Mom was also a very good cook, but I never learned much about cooking at home. Maybe she tried to teach me, but I just wasn't interested. When I got to eighth grade, all the girls had to take home economics. The classroom overlooked the tennis courts, so there I was, cooking, and just hating it because I wanted to be outside playing tennis. The first thing I had to cook was lentil soup—and I hated lentils! Well, I made the soup anyway, and of course, I had to taste it. I ended up liking it. Now I love lentils, and I make a special lentil salad that is absolutely delicious.

I actually love to cook now, and I'm pretty good at it. Back in 1976, I knew I had a talent for cooking when my team tennis roommate in Cleveland, Wendy Overton, taught me how to make an omelet. Hers broke. Mine didn't. I was thus on my way to becoming a chef extraordinaire! Okay, so I'm exaggerating a bit. But come over for dinner at Chez Martina, and you will be asking for seconds.

THE UPS AND DOWNS OF MY WEIGHT

Like most of you, I've had weight fluctuations, and I do have to watch what I eat. When I first came to America in 1973 at the age of 16, I put on 20 pounds in 2 weeks. Back then, reporters wrote that my parents didn't recognize me, but that wasn't exactly true. They could recognize *me;* they just couldn't recognize the other 20 pounds.

That was also when my metabolism was changing due to puberty. Meals in America were protein, protein, and more protein. In the Czech Republic, we ate mostly carbohydrates, with a small amount of protein. Here, I'd have a huge steak for dinner, along with a baked potato, a salad, soup—and two scoops of ice cream every night for dessert. My metabolism just couldn't get all that stuff organized, particularly the meat, and it went straight to my waistline and jowls. Protein and puberty—I just ballooned because of that pairing.

For a few years, I didn't lose that initial weight, even though I tried to play myself into shape. I eventually shot up to my heaviest, around 170 pounds, in January 1976. I just didn't know enough about a healthy diet back then. I kept playing and eating. Finally, at the end of 1976, the weight came off pretty much on its own. I guess my baby fat days were over. Since then, my weight has stabilized at around 145. However, it was only in 1981 that I realized it's the lean muscular quality of the 145 pounds that really counts. That's when I went to a diet of pasta, grains, salads, fruits, and lean protein and laid off the animal fats, sugar, and processed foods. A skin-fold caliper test showed that my total weight was only 8.8 percent body fat, compared to the average 12 to 14 percent for tennis players. I felt like a new person.

Another time—in 1993—I put on weight

because I couldn't say no to dessert. I was just eating far too much. I thought, "No problem. Once I start working out, the weight will come off." Can you believe it? The first day back at training, I badly sprained my right ankle and was laid up for another month, and I kept eating. When the buttons were about to pop off my clothes, I had another one of those heart-to-self talks. "Self," I said, "this can't go on, or else I'll look like I did in the seventies." I knew I wouldn't be able to function on or off the court, either, and my extra weight was going to place undue stress on my already weakened ankle. So I got my diet under control. I stopped eating so much volume. I cut out desserts for a few weeks and gradually lost the weight. I was still 10 pounds overweight at the Italian Open, but 6 weeks later, by Wimbledon, I was back to my normal weight of 145. You live and learn.

That was also when I started to use a belt to monitor the ups and downs in my weight. I still have that belt. It is thick and doesn't stretch, so I know exactly which notch it should be on when I'm at a good, healthy weight. If I go up a notch or more, I know I've got to get in gear and course-correct—which means paying attention to what I eat, easing down on the volume a bit, and working out a little harder. I want to perform as well as I can—and feel good while performing. But I can't do that if I'm eating junk and weighing in at too much over my normal weight.

The only other time that I had issues with my weight was after I retired from singles competition in 1994, in a rather tearful farewell at Madison Square Garden. I couldn't play myself into shape because I was playing hardly any

tennis. I wasn't training on a regular basis—hardly at all, in fact. I ate as I pleased, and a lot of that food wasn't burned off. It just settled in.

LIFE IN RETIREMENT

With retirement, I had the freedom to do whatever I wanted—and I did. I learned to fly a plane and got my pilot's license. It was fantastic. Flying is the ultimate form of freedom—as long as there's gas in the tank, of course.

I also took a few woodworking classes, and as a budding carpenter, I designed and built two tables. I had more time for political activism and was one of the speakers at the 2000 Millennium March in Washington, D.C. I traveled to Kenya, my favorite spot in the whole world, and spent 5 months there on two separate trips. I observed and photographed elephants, lions, and all kinds of animals and birds in the African bush. I spent more time with my family and friends. And I didn't miss tennis.

I remember one year during my retirement, I was vacationing on a houseboat on Lake Powell, a man-made lake formed when Glen Canyon Dam backed up the waters of the Colorado and San Juan rivers. Few places on Earth have such exquisite natural beauty (with or without the water that fills the canyon). The lake is bordered by beautiful side canyons, colorful rock walls, natural domes and arches, and remnants of ancient Indian cultures. Indian legend has it that if you pray while passing under one of the arches, called the Rainbow Bridge, you'll cast your troubles aside. That's certainly how I felt—trouble-free. During that vacation, the U.S. Open was going on, but I didn't know who won until I got home the following Wednesday. And frankly, I didn't care. I was happy not doing anything, even happy not playing tennis. I felt that if I didn't pick up a racquet for the rest of my life, I'd be happy.

I was wrong, though. I did pick up a racquet, and I didn't want to put it down again. I officially returned to doubles competition in 2000. Part of what moved me to "get back in the game" was my weight—not the desire to beat anyone's records, as has been rumored. As I mentioned, I had gotten a little heavy while retired and felt very sluggish. I hated that feeling, so I started training to get back in shape. Each year after I quit playing, I had done TV commentary at Wimbledon, yet I had no desire to play again. But in 1999, for some reason, I said to myself, "What the heck? I've gotten in good shape. Why not play doubles?" And I thought, "Maybe next year."

When my good friend, South African Mariaan de Swardt, who had played on the tour but had been injured for some time, asked me in March of 2000 if I would be interested in playing Wimbledon with her that year, I said, "Sure!" Little did I know that 1 year would turn into many more years of playing.

We played a succession of tournaments— the Madrid Open, the French Open, and Eastbourne—all leading up to Wimbledon, where we won three matches and got to the quarterfinals before losing to the Sisters Sledgehammer, Serena and Venus Williams. As it turned out, we were the only team that took a set from them. The amazing response from the fans, the media, and my peers was such that I didn't want to stop. People were saying how inspired they were. Teenagers said things like, "Hey, Martina, you rock."

I realized I could still hang with the younger tennis players on the tour. I could beat some of them in singles, and I could beat most of them in doubles. So why not? The ball doesn't know how old I am.

In January 2003, I went on to win the Australian Open mixed doubles title with my doubles partner, Leander Paes. That victory, at age 46, made me the oldest winner, male or female, of a Grand Slam title. Funny, isn't it? When I was growing up, I wanted to be the youngest to win something—not the oldest!

THE OLDEST TENNIS PLAYER IN THE HISTORY OF THE OLYMPICS

When I started my comeback at the age of 43, never did I realize that getting in great shape athletically would ultimately result in being selected to represent the United States at the Olympics in Athens 4 years later, in 2004. Playing in the Olympics meant everything to me. It was one of the few sporting events in which I had never had the opportunity to compete as a tennis player. I missed the 1988, 1992, 1996, and 2000 Olympics for a variety of reasons, mainly burnout, contractual commitments, and retirement. When it became realistic for me to play in the Olympics, I set my sights on it in 2004. I adjusted my schedule. I teamed up with another American, Lisa Raymond, so that we could potentially go to the Olympics together as a team. I played solid, passionate tennis that year. It paid off. I earned the honor of playing in the Olympics by being one of the top four doubles players in America—at age 47! When I finally got there, I turned out to be the oldest Olympic tennis player in the history of the Games, eclipsing the mark set at the 1924 Paris Games by 46-year-old Australian Norman Brookes.

At the Olympics, I was thinking of all the opening ceremonies I had ever watched, plus all the Games. I don't think any American athlete can have a greater thrill than to stand there at those ceremonies wearing the same uniform as your teammates, proud to represent the United States. It was just amazing to be there and to be touched by the Olympic spirit.

The first ball I tossed up to serve, I thought, "Hey, this is your first Olympic toss." It was a good one. I looked around. Everyone looked about 12 years old. That confirmed it: Yes, I was the oldest athlete there!

My hopes for a medal were dashed, though, when Lisa and I lost in a hard-fought quarterfinal match against Japan. Even so, competing in the Olympics was a wonderful new experience, the experience of a lifetime. I loved it. I wouldn't have passed it up for anything.

The way I see it, you never regret new experiences, only the ones you've missed.

FROM ME TO YOU

My hope for you is that this book becomes one of those new experiences, something that enlightens you and empowers you toward real change. My goal in writing it is to echo the voice that may be whispering inside you—the voice urging you on to real lifestyle change—and to support your decision on every page. I will say up front that I do not aim to win a grammar contest with my sentence structure. Nope, I'm not out to win grammar contests, but what I'm trying to do is share my thoughts with each and every one of you who choose to pick up this book.

Our world is filled with people from so many walks of life that it would be literally impossible to meet and discuss our individual definitions of what it means to have a healthy lifestyle. But think about what led you to this book. Who are you, and what is driving you? It is important to reflect upon who we are really, on the inside as well as the outside. That is how I believe transformation starts, from the inside, deep down inside.

Have you ever walked around a bookstore or library and noticed the amazing amount of books on health and fitness? I especially like titles such as *How to Eat Your Way to Good Health* or *The Miracle Way to a New You* or, better still, *The Only Diet Book You'll Ever Need—Ever!* Honestly, sometimes I think the people writing these books are alumni of the same college—Know-It-All U. I have a friend who knows a great deal about many things, yet ask her a question, and she will always say, "I don't have all the answers but . . ." I can honestly say that 99 percent of the time my friend does in fact have the answer, but if she doesn't, she does research to get it. She never makes others feel less than what or who they are. On the contrary, she makes them participate in the discovery of the answer. That is how I would like to approach my effort to help encourage and support your lifestyle change. I don't have all the answers, but I have some ideas as to how to approach changes that will make you think and, hopefully, start with baby steps toward changes that will make a real difference in your tomorrow.

Please don't just pick up this book, read it cover to cover, and then jump into change. Read the book, put it down, reflect upon its purpose, then pick it up again and again and even again. Consider where you are today and why you bought this book. If it was because I'm a sports figure, then thank you for picking it up, but be honest, maybe that alone wasn't the reason. Maybe you are a person who wants to make real changes in your life. If so, I'm thrilled that I can help you in some way on your journey to better health and fitness.

Throughout this book, I will share my personal experiences and those of people from my past and present. I will share how we have all taken steps toward healthy lifestyle changes. These changes were very realistic for a few of them, but others went to the extreme and then needed a reality check to figure out that the change was only a quick fix and not realistic or lasting.

FINISH STRONG

My wish for you is that you make shaping your self a project that you finish. Far too many people start projects but never complete them. They think they are too difficult. The projects take too much time. They forget about them. Or they meet obstacles they feel they can't overcome, and so they wander off the path.

Let me tell you a story: One of my heroes and role models is Katharine Hepburn. I've been a Hepburn fan ever since I saw her in *The*

African Queen when I was a child. It was one of the first American films I ever saw. From then on, I wanted to be like Katharine Hepburn, and my big hope was to meet her someday. Once, I sent her flowers on her birthday and included my address on the card. She wrote back, thanking me for the flowers and inviting me for a visit if I was ever in New York City. Two months later, I got up enough nerve to call her. She answered on the second ring. I recognized her distinctive voice right away.

"Miss Hepburn, this is Martina Navratilova."

"It's about time," she said.

Those were her first words to me.

So I visited her at her apartment in New York City, the first of many visits over the years. Katharine Hepburn was exactly the way I had imagined: so much style, such poise, as bright as could be, and so, so curious—more interested in other people than in herself. She had more wisdom than anyone else I had ever met. She once told me something I've never forgotten: "It's not what you start in life, it's what you finish." Those words became a guiding creed for me.

What about you? Will you make the final push and finish what you start?

I began this Introduction talking about questions people ask me these days. I'd like to close it with one other question they ask now that I've hit midlife: "Why are you still playing?" My answer: "Because I can."

But more than that, you can, too. Young or old, you *can* achieve the shape of your life.

I did it. So can you. I may be a well-known professional tennis player, with advantages afforded by my fame. But fame doesn't exempt you from any of life's normal problems and issues. It just means you can't lose your cool in public without reading about it in the newspaper the next day. Like you, I have ups and downs and trials and triumphs. Most of us have great lives, really, or at least the opportunity to have great lives, so why not go forward with a positive attitude, enjoy life to the fullest, and make the most of it?

That's my hope for you. I'd like to get you started on making the most of your life by sharing with you everything I know about doing it. The ability to share what I have—whether it's information or a possession—is something I got from my beloved Grandma Subertova, the most generous person I have ever known. What made her happy was making other people happy. One of her favorite ways of making me happy was to make me her special carrot salad. "Eat it," she'd say. "It's good for your eyes. You will see the ball better."

When I was a little kid in school, if I took an orange for lunch—and oranges weren't easy to come by in the Czech Republic—I'd always give the bigger part to a friend. I understood early on that it is better to give than to receive.

I know that getting your body, your health, and your life in shape isn't easy. But if you take at least half of what I have to share with you, you will get there. Like so many people who believed in me over the years and gave me my chance in tennis, I believe in you. Now, here's your chance to get in the shape of your life.

STEPS TO SHAPE
YOUR SELF

I once had a coach, Mike Estep, who challenged a lot of the patterns that I had picked up in my first decade on the women's tour. I had developed a tendency to hit from the baseline, for example, rather than act on my natural impulse to rush the net. Mike broke down a lot of those patterns, working with what I had, to help me become better.

That's exactly what I'd like to do for you in this first part of the book: help break down habitual patterns that can jeopardize your health and well-being. The six steps you are about to learn are the gateway to doing that. Let them form the strategy you will need to get in the shape of your life.

Mike always used to say, "Charge; take a little chance," and I say the same to you. Take a chance. Doing things differently and better is what it's all about.

CHAPTER 1

MAKE YOUR OWN
COMEBACK

This is your life. Do the most you can with it.

A letter that I will never forget arrived in the mail one day. Every time I think about it, my eyes well up with tears. The letter was written by a woman who had been confined to a wheelchair for years due to a crippling muscle disease. She had read about my comeback from retirement, and it inspired her to such a level that she began to see new possibilities for herself. Something inside her burst open, gathered strength, and gushed out in the form of desire: desire to break free and walk again, desire to play her favorite sport—tennis—once again. Inspired, she directed the full force of her energy to make her own comeback. She got out of her wheelchair and fulfilled her desires.

What about you? Do you need to make a comeback—perhaps from poor health, an out-of-shape body, a bad attitude, or shattered self-confidence? I bring up this story to tell you that all things are possible when you have the desire to change and approach it with a self-loving attitude. You can make your own comeback, too.

MAKE THE CHOICE

From the day we are born, most of us bounce into this world healthy. Then something goes wrong. That "something" is us. We begin to habitually make poor health choices. We eat mass-produced junk food that is toxic to our bodies. We veg out on the couch, even though our bodies were designed to move. We gain weight that our bodies were never intended to lug around. We smoke, drink too much alcohol, or do drugs, taking in poisons that irreparably damage the integrity of our cells.

As humans living in industrialized countries today, we're far off the mark from the lifestyle that we were meant to live. The outermost sign of this is our physical shape: pounds and pounds of fat that mar the natural beauty of the human form, gravely interfere with our normal activities, lessen our quality of life, hurt our financial situations, and, of course, shorten our life spans.

The way I see it, people are just not meant to be overweight. To anyone who's overweight and claims to be happy, I'd say, "What planet are you living on? Who are you trying to convince—me or yourself?"

On planet Earth, America is the fattest of all nations; the number of obese people is staggering, despite all the low-fat foods, low-carb products, diet drinks, and artificial sweeteners we consume. (In fact, you have to search high and low to find full-fat yogurt, which is what I like.) With all these diet foods around, it's hard to figure why so many people are overweight.

By contrast, in Europe, you would be hard-pressed to find severely overweight people, and in Africa, where I've traveled and lived, you seldom see people with weight problems. They work hard just to eke out a living and put food on the table, so there's little opportunity to overindulge.

In many respects, they're like our ancestors, the early hunters and gatherers who hunted wild game and collected plant foods to eat. During times of plenty, their bodies were designed to store food as fat to be used as fuel during periods of famine. As their descendants, we inherited this ability to store fat. However, there are no famines in America these days, so the fat we store is not burned but continues to accrue through the years. We no longer hunt and collect as our forebears did. Instead, we pop food in the microwave or get it at the drive-thru, then just collect it in our bellies.

From what I understand, the natural diet of our ancestors served them well. Archaeological records reveal that they lived relatively free of heart disease, cancer, hypertension, diabetes, osteoporosis, and other diseases that are killing us off today. Many nutritionists and scientists feel that we're genetically programmed to thrive on a diet of natural foods—fruits, vegetables, nuts, seeds, grains, and low-fat meats—just as our ancestors did. I believe them. It just makes sense, this evolutionary inheritance that resides in us. But the problem is that we pollute our bodies with cheeseburgers, sodas, potato chips, and candy bars. It's no wonder our bodies break down and get so sick: We're feeding them foods they register as poisons.

You've probably read the same statistics I have: In the United States alone, poor diets and physical inactivity account for more than 400,000 deaths each year. Smoking kills approximately 440,000 people yearly. Wouldn't you say we're choosing a suicidal lifestyle?

By choosing differently, taking better care of yourself and making healthy choices, you increase your odds of preventing, and even reversing, life-threatening illnesses. And who knows? You may live to be 100 or even more, still vital, still in robust health. I don't know about you, but I intend to die at a very *healthy* old age.

If you start following just some of the tips and guidelines here, at the very least, you'll start looking and feeling better right away. If you do them all, there's no telling how much better you will feel and look, and there's no telling how much better and healthier you will live. Let me ask you: When was the last time you felt really healthy? Energetic? Attractive? In charge of your mind and your mood?

One thing you can definitely control is the shape of your life. It's your choice. From what I've read and been told, the biggest influences on your health are diet, behavior, and environment. You can control your diet. You can control your behavior. And to a large extent, you can control your environment. But what about your genes? Isn't a lot of disease a result of what's been passed on to you by your parents? Not necessarily, say many health experts. Genes rarely cause disease; they just make us more susceptible to certain types. I've heard genetics described as a loaded gun; bad health choices simply pull the trigger. Your body is a self-healing, self-governing system that will maintain good health if you give it the right nutrients, the right amount of activity, the right emotional balance—in short, the right care. In other words, give your body a chance!

Maybe you've been telling yourself, "I've got to do something," but you don't know how to go about it. That's why I've created this easy-to-follow six-step program. My former coach Mike Estep used to say, "Tennis is a lot like chess, but a lot of women are playing without a couple of pieces. Some of them can't hit an overhead or a topspin forehand. Martina happens to have all the pieces on the board."

Maybe you've been trying to get in shape, but until now, you haven't had all the pieces available to you. To shape your self, you must have all the pieces on the board—everything you need working in sync to tune up your body, mind, and spirit. These six steps are those pieces.

So what are they? The steps are based on strategies I've used over the years—a lifestyle I've designed for myself, based partly on good sense and largely on scientific soundness. It isn't a fad; it's a way of life. It was a long time coming, too. When I started out, for example, people used to think that steak and eggs was a good meal to eat before a match. Everyone was pretty clueless about nutrition and training back then. With all that I've learned about food, exercise, and health, I just wish I could have put these strategies to use much earlier in my career. But better late than never.

Here's an overview of Part 1—the six steps—and Part 2—the Shape Your Self nutrition and exercise plans.

PART 1: STEPS TO SHAPE YOUR SELF

Step 1: Develop the Mentality of an Athlete

When I was about 7, my father used to say, "Make believe you're at Wimbledon." So, in my mind's eye, I'd see myself standing at

Centre Court, holding up my trophy. He planted those kinds of dreams in me, and as I grew up, I began to dream on my own.

Those dreams gelled into what is called an athlete's mentality—an attitude, a mind-set, a singleness of purpose to become the best that you can. It's formed in your heart and mind, and it becomes part of who you are. More practically, it involves goal-setting and using logs or journals to monitor performance, provide feedback, and see if any patterns, good or bad, are emerging.

You don't have to be an athlete to develop an athlete's mentality. You can use the same techniques to develop a sense of discipline, focus, and purpose that will take you to the top in every part of your life. I'll show you those techniques in this step so you can build up your inner strength and good health.

Step 2: Build Your Support Team

I believe in having a support system for whatever you do. It gives you the strength to keep going. I've always had a few of my friends and advisors sit together and cheer for me during a match, a coach or trainer who helped me play up to my potential, or a friend who might say, "Come on; snap out of it" when my moods are as overcast as a cloudy day. Companionship was something I got used to when I was 13, having teammates I played tennis with. I wasn't just out there for myself—and that was fun. The bond formed with teammates lasts a lifetime.

With the encouragement and support of others, your efforts will start to pick up immediately. When people are there for you, you want to be with them. At the emotional level, there's a certain feeling of fulfillment that comes from being around people you like and who like you. They hold you together when you feel like you're falling apart. Even research shows that people with support systems are more likely to make healthier choices, experience less depression, and live longer.

Your support system can keep watch over you, too, to help you kick your bad habits and put some control in your life. I remember that back in the eighties, one of the habits I had gotten into was buying something for myself whenever I was feeling down—expensive toys like cars and jewelry. I'd go on these spending binges to compensate for losing.

At that time, basketball great Nancy Lieberman, who was playing with the Dallas Diamonds of the Women's Basketball League, was training me. Back then, she set me straight on my spending habits. "You've got it all wrong," she told me. "You don't buy something because you lost a tournament and you want to feel good about yourself. You buy something because you want it and you deserve it. You don't deserve something for losing. You have to earn it."

I came to realize that habitual spending could become as destructive as relying on drugs and alcohol, overeating, or starving yourself. We all have a negative escape hatch somewhere! Had it not been for Nancy lighting into me like that, it may have taken me a lot longer to get the wake-up call I needed.

So in this step, we'll talk about how you can build a positive network of people as well as what to do when relationships become counterproductive. Unless your support system has a positive influence on you, it can be tough to reach the goals you set for yourself.

Step 3: Fuel Your Body and Mind

Good nutrition is the foundation of performance in every area of an active, successful life. In this step, you'll learn how to introduce natural foods, including raw foods and juices, into your diet. Trust me, as soon as you try this way of eating, you'll be able to feel the difference it makes in your body. You'll feel so much lighter and so much stronger without a lot of unnatural substances in your body. You'll start feeling more vibrant. Your body will release toxins. You'll automatically lose weight if you need to. Your skin will look more youthful (an outward sign of inner rejuvenation). You'll experience boundless energy. And you'll think more clearly and creatively.

I attribute the ageless way I feel now to how I eat, and I see no reason why I won't feel this great well into my golden years. It has made that much of a difference. You'll be able to execute this food plan easily and even cheat on it occasionally. Yes, it's okay—indeed, it's healthy—to cheat every now and then. I don't believe in overdoing anything.

Step 4: Go Organic

Today, we have access to a plethora of food sources: raw, canned, bottled, boxed, vacuum sealed, and even freeze dried. We have quantity, but quality is what we've sacrificed over the past 50 years, and as a result, life-threatening illnesses have surfaced with a vengeance and at a rate that is alarming.

In this step, I'll talk about how buying organic foods is one of the ways you can ensure the quality of the food you serve. Organic fruits, vegetables, and grains are grown without the use of most conventional pesticides and without fertilizers made with synthetic ingredients. Organic meats and dairy products are free of antibiotics and growth hormones.

Maybe you haven't gone organic yet because you think the food is too expensive. You're right; it can be. But I've found that shopping around pays off. Places like specialty stores, co-ops, gourmet delis, farmers' markets, and community-supported agricultural programs sell organic foods that are economically priced. The one thing I'm thankful for is that there are so many places where I can buy organic produce and other foods. Fortunately, with the growing demand, prices are coming down.

There are other ways to go organic, too, besides the food you eat. This is where I'll also talk about how to eliminate pollutants from your personal environment with organic alternatives and safer solutions. Did you know, for example, that you don't have to spray chemical pesticides in your house to kill bugs, that red chili powder can get rid of ants, or that chopped bay leaves and cucumber skins can repel other pests? There are so many positive benefits to your health that can be achieved by creating a less toxic environment for yourself, inside and out.

Step 5: Build the Fitness to Function

I never did like conventional exercises—you know, like repetitive calisthenics. In grade school, I'd go to any length to avoid them. Can you relate? But if exercise has a lot of mix-it-up variety in it (I have a short attention span), I'm game.

The techniques you'll learn in this step are fun, unique, and cutting edge. You can do these simple yet challenging workouts at home with just a few inexpensive and easy-to-store pieces of equipment. You don't even need a gym membership.

My exercises target body parts you want to overhaul. They focus on strength and cardio. They're designed to develop your energy system and rejuvenate your body. Whether you're a beginner at exercise or have some experience already, I will meet you where you are. I'll show you how to challenge yourself depending on your level of conditioning. I promise that this is one approach to exercise with which you will not get bored. I don't know about you, but I like to concentrate and think about what I'm doing when I work out. I want to be aware of my body and what it's trying to do, not just "get through it." So I'll guide you through some focusing techniques that will make you appreciate the power, strength, and beauty of your body and what it's capable of doing.

This kind of training, coupled with good nutrition, has helped me be in the best shape of my career. I know it has made me stronger than other women on the court and faster than most, but not bigger than a lot of them. In fact, the conditioning exercises will help you reshape areas of your body where you want better, or different, contours.

With the training I do, form follows function. In other words, I train specifically so that I can functionally improve my tennis. You can train that way, too—for a specific sport—or you can train for a better look, such as a better-shaped butt, toned arms, a flatter belly, longer muscles, or all of the above. It's up to you, and my exercise guidelines give you the flexibility to meet your personal fitness goals. You'll look better, and you'll perform better in whatever you need to do. You'll feel healthy and be bursting with confidence. And that confidence will show.

Step 6: Recharge and Energize—When You're Tired of Being Tired

When I was first inspired to write this book, I knew immediately that I wanted to do a chapter asking: Are you tired of being tired? I know I was! I've been in too many situations, on and off the court, in which I didn't have as much energy as I would have liked. If I feel wiped out when I'm playing or training, I could put stress on my body. I could hurt a knee or a shoulder or an ankle by falling, not to mention lose a match. When I'm exhausted, I don't have enough stamina to do a lot of the activities and sports I enjoy. I've always liked to test the limits of my body while it's still capable of pushing the limits. I want to know exactly where that limit is and keep pushing it. After all, the only way to not fail in anything is to do nothing.

Over the years, I've learned to listen to my body, paying attention to its cries for help, and let it dictate the right pace so I don't experience fatigue. Here's where I'll share with you my techniques for recharging. You'll find out how to be a better steward of your own energy system and how to boost your energy production to meet your body's demands.

PART 2: THE SHAPE YOUR SELF NUTRITION AND EXERCISE PLANS

The second part of the book "puts it all to-gether" for you. It introduces you to a healthy meal plan that will manage your nutrition for better health. This is based on the way I eat, and it has helped keep my body in peak condi-tion and working well. If you follow the menus pretty closely, you should soon start looking and feeling better.

Next is a fitness section where you'll learn dozens of fun exercises designed for different levels of fitness. These exercises are a part of my own routine. Until several years ago, I was never really aware that there are so many new exercises you can do to get fit. My trainers began to teach me new moves, and this new knowledge about exercising was challenging and exciting. It's always fun for me to learn new ways to exercise. I like to move and I like to be challenged, and these exercises help me do that. Together, both of these sections offer you some great tools to get in shape and stay that way.

CHANGING THE SHAPE OF YOUR LIFE

To attain the shape of your life, I believe you must be open to change—changing a habit, a pattern of behavior, an attitude, a way of liv-ing—but do it gradually. I think people can handle change better if it's gradual and if they don't have blind spots when it comes to what needs changing.

Studies have shown, however, that people are generally resistant to change. It makes them feel uncomfortable, out of sync. Bottom line:

Change frightens them. Most people like rou-tine. How many times have you heard someone say, "I wish things could be the way they used to be" or "I like things just the way they are"?

Sometimes, though, we just have to pause and take inventory. If you honestly look over the areas of your life that call out for change, what concerns you the most about your lifestyle? Is it poor nutrition? Lack of exercise? Being tired all the time? Putting on weight be-cause you're eating poorly? Being too busy to enjoy life? Needing to carve out more time for rest and relaxation? Rearranging priorities? Retrospection, and introspection, are all about pausing and taking inventory of ourselves. Read through "Your Personal Health and Fitness Inventory" on page 10. It may alert you to factors in your life that are positively or neg-atively affecting your health. Simply circle yes or no for each question, then study what your answers mean.

TIME FOR A CHANGE

Sure, change is difficult, but it allows us to be better than we were or ever knew we could be. It's the gateway to personal growth and new ex-periences. Unless we change, we keep repeating the same mistakes. You know this yourself if you've ever lost weight and regained it, over and over again.

Many people don't want to retool their lifestyles because their fear of failure is too great. Are you like that? You don't even get going on a quest because you're afraid you won't make it? But if you're afraid of some-thing, you won't change anything.

(continued on page 13)

YOUR PERSONAL HEALTH AND FITNESS INVENTORY

1. Do you try to eat at least 5 servings of fruits and vegetables each day?

   Yes   No

2. Do you try to limit your consumption of red meat to a few times a month?

   Yes   No

3. Do you eat mostly natural carbohydrates, such as whole grains, instead of processed carbs, such as sweets?

   Yes   No

4. Do you try to limit your intake of foods containing additives, preservatives, or artificial colors?

   Yes   No

5. Do you ever buy organically grown foods?

   Yes   No

6. Do you drink at least 8 cups of pure water daily?

   Yes   No

7. Do you try to limit your consumption of soft drinks, including diet sodas?

   Yes   No

8. Are you happy, or comfortable, with your present weight?

   Yes   No

9. Do you limit your intake of alcoholic beverages to one or two drinks daily or have none at all?

   Yes   No

10. Do you limit your intake of coffee and caffeine-containing beverages to 1 serving a day or have none at all?

    Yes   No

11. Do you exercise for 30 minutes or more at least three times a week?

    Yes   No

12. Do you regularly participate in stress-reducing activities, such as relaxation, meditation, reading, exercise, yoga, hobbies, or other fun activities?

    Yes   No

13. Do you get enough satisfying sleep most nights of the week?

    Yes   No

14. Are you a nonsmoker, or if you used to smoke cigarettes, have you quit?

    Yes   No

15. Do you have a supportive network of friends and family to whom you are connected?

    Yes   No

What Your Responses May Mean

For every yes you circled, take credit for your healthy habits and congratulate yourself. You've already accomplished a lot more than you realize. Reflect on the things you're doing right and vow to continue them. The nos you circled simply mean you have work to do in some areas. We all do. I remember when one of my coaches told me I could be the greatest female player ever, but I wasn't playing up to my potential. I was in good physical and emotional shape, but my strategic game left a lot to be desired. There's always room for improvement.

Here's a closer look at what your responses mean, question by question.

1. If you're eating fewer than 5 servings of these foods, you're skimping on a lot of healthy, anti-aging nutrients. Green

veggies, for example, are loaded with folate, a nutrient that reduces the risk of common aging-related diseases. Fresh produce is rich in antioxidants, which are thought to prevent harm to our cells caused by destructive chemicals called free radicals. For great health and rejuvenation, fruits and vegetables need to be the centerpiece of your diet.

2. Too much red meat in the diet can be hard on your body. It's high in saturated fat, which can contribute to blocked arteries, and a diet overloaded with red meat has been implicated in colon cancer. For a lot of people, it's hard to digest. The digestive system slows with age, so I think it's better to curb your intake of red meat, especially as you get older. If you enjoy eating it, just try to make it a treat by having it only a few times a month.

3. I hope you answered yes. If you did, you've said no to a group of foods—sugar and processed foods—that are rough on your metabolism. Eating these foods throws your blood sugar out of whack, and you're apt to feel tired and hungry as a result of blood sugar levels going up and down. What's more, these foods have very little fiber, so they don't contribute much to the 20 to 35 grams that you need daily for good health. Whole grains give you plenty of fiber, plus B vitamins, which defend your heart and brain from age-related diseases.

4. Processed foods, as opposed to natural, whole foods, have a lot of stuff added to them—stuff that supplies very little, if any, nutrition. Additives, preservatives, and artificial colors in foods have been linked to allergies and disease, so it's best to choose additive-free, natural foods whenever you can.

5. Organic foods are those produced without pesticides, hormones, or antibiotics. These foods have been shown to be higher in nutrients and are a better all-around choice for ensuring the quality of your diet. Say yes to organic!

6. Drinking ample water throughout the day is a great habit if you want to stay healthy and lean (water aids in metabolism) and feel youthful. Very often, feeling tired during the day is a sign that you're dehydrated.

7. Drinking sodas when you're thirsty can really rack up the calories and promote weight gain. Soft drinks are loaded with sugar—about 10 teaspoons per can—and are among the worst beverage choices. Even if you drink diet soda, your body gets confused by the artificial sweeteners in it, according to research. For some sugar-sensitive people, diet sodas may stimulate cravings for more sweets. They may also elevate blood sugar in the same way regular soda does. When your blood sugar goes up sharply, your body releases insulin, a hormone that tells your body to store calories as fat.

8. If you're not happy with your weight, maybe you're overweight and perhaps at risk of obesity. Being heavy is more than an appearance issue. Obesity puts you at risk for developing one or more serious medical conditions, which can cause poor health and prema-

(cont.)

ture death. In fact, obesity is associated with more than 30 medical conditions. Among the short list of obesity-related ills are heart disease, type 2 diabetes, certain cancers, and kidney disease. (A lot of people think they're fat even when their doctors tell them they're within a healthy weight range. If you fit that description, it may mean you have a body image problem that needs to be sorted out through counseling.)

9. Despite some of the health claims attributed to alcohol, it can be detrimental to your body. Excessive alcohol consumption promotes weight gain, dehydrates your body, can be addictive, contributes too much sugar and few nutrients, and can lead to organ damage. It's best to monitor your intake or switch to nonalcoholic drinks.

10. Caffeine is a powerful stimulant found in coffee, tea, soft drinks, and many over-the-counter medicines. If you're having trouble falling asleep or staying asleep, limit your intake to one or two cups of coffee in the morning or eliminate caffeine altogether. Anyone who has heart disease, an irregular heartbeat, or high blood pressure should avoid caffeine altogether, since it elevates stress hormones that can have harmful effects on the cardiovascular system. If you want to reduce your caffeine intake, switch to green tea. It's loaded with disease-fighting, anti-aging antioxidants.

11. Exercising on a regular basis drastically cuts the risk of high blood pressure and stroke. It also helps you lose weight and maintain that weight loss. Regular exercise slows bone loss, eases anxiety and stress, boosts immunity, improves sleep, and lowers the risk of type 2 diabetes.

12. Rest and relaxation will keep you young! Beyond its well-known connection to heart disease and high blood pressure, stress—even a little bit—can harm your concentration and memory. Stress-reducing activities like those listed in this question can clear your mind and ease your body.

13. There's a reason it's called beauty sleep! Anti-aging hormones such as melatonin, human growth hormone, and testosterone are produced in greater amounts at night during sleep. When you don't get enough sleep, your body isn't able to make these hormones in the amounts it needs. Also, lack of sleep can cause the release of a stress hormone called cortisol, which, according to a lot of studies, is directly tied to weight gain. To feel and look your best, you need 7 to 9 hours of good sleep each night.

14. I've read that quitting smoking can add nearly 9 years to your life span. I believe it. Smoking is estimated to cause one-third of all cancer deaths and one-fourth of fatal heart attacks in the United States. Approximately 440,000 Americans die each year from diseases related to smoking, according to the American Lung Association.

15. Stay connected with friends and loved ones. A large number of studies suggests that continuing close relationships into old age has a positive impact on your health.

Or maybe you're a born procrastinator. Okay, I'll admit it, so am I—or I was. Procrastination is an old habit that many times in my life kept winning out. I'd let problems slide and slide, mostly because I needed shelter from them when I was playing tennis. Conflict, for example—I tried to avoid it at all costs. I would just let things build, and they'd get worse. But just imagine what might happen if you let your health slide. Who wants to hear a doctor say, "If you don't stop smoking, you'll be dead in 6 months" or "If you don't stop drinking, your liver will give out in 2 years"? Don't let things deteriorate into a life-or-death situation. Please! I learned to deal with problems head on, and sooner rather than later. You can as well.

One important rule in this process is to make meaningful changes that you want for you, not for others. Changes made to please others are unrealistic, but more important, they're unfair to you.

You've heard the cliché about how a journey begins with a single step? The journey to shape your self unfolds incrementally. All I ask is that you take a single step, then another one, then another. Just put one foot in front of the other and don't worry about the length of the path. Once you get on that path, and the longer you stay on it, there eventually will come a time when you will not turn back. You'll be on the path to good health the rest of your life.

The key word is *gradual*. For years, a good friend of mine tried to quit smoking. She was never successful until she decided to take a gradual approach. She told herself, "I'm not going to smoke in the car." She stopped smoking in the car. Next, she said, "I'm not going to smoke in the bedroom." She stopped smoking in the bedroom. Then she vowed, "I'm not going to smoke when I'm on the phone." That was a tough one for her. Whenever the phone rang, it was like a signal to smoke, and she lit up a cigarette without thinking. But she was able to stop her automatic behavior. At that point, she was down to about three cigarettes a day and ultimately was able to quit. You see, she gradually and systematically eliminated every habitual circumstance that caused her to light up.

You might do the same. Think long term and don't go for the quick fix. Just take it day by day. Perhaps start by giving yourself at least a half hour each day to take care of yourself in some way. Before you know it, you've lost 5 pounds or lowered your blood pressure or stopped drinking or smoking. You start feeling a difference. You start looking better, without expensive creams or makeovers. You turn heads, with people wondering why you look so great and how you did it. Your new, more vibrant health shines through from the inside, and that to me is exciting.

Something I read recently made a huge impression on me, and I want to share it with you before we move on. It is from a book titled *How to Think like Leonardo da Vinci* by Michael J. Gelb (Bantam Dell, 1998). In it, Gelb lists Leonardo's personal rules for staying healthy. Here are some of them.

- Beware of anger and avoid grievous moods.
- Rest your head and keep your mind cheerful.
- Be covered well at night.
- Exercise moderately.
- Shun wantonness and pay attention to diet.

- Eat only when you want and sup light.
- Let your wine be mixed with water, take a little at a time, not between meals and not on an empty stomach.
- Eat simple food.
- Chew well.
- Go to the toilet regularly!

Those are some simple yet very powerful thoughts from one of history's true Renaissance men, who, like many health advocates today, believed in a holistic philosophy of health and medicine. To me, Da Vinci had more talents and smarts than any human who ever lived. By following just a few principles of healthful living like those listed above, you can make some pretty dramatic improvements in your own well-being.

THE PURSUIT OF EXCELLENCE

Let me emphasize that getting in shape is not about the pursuit of perfection. It's about the pursuit of excellence. You can be excellent without being perfect, and that's the key. Excellence doesn't involve trying to be the best; it means making your best effort in whatever you do.

Perfection is very elusive and really nonexistent. It can lead to disappointment. Trying to attain perfection, whether it's the perfect body or the perfect performance, can also wear you down physically and emotionally. That's because the stress and worry of trying to be perfect can actually decrease mood-lifting chemicals and deplete glucose levels in your

brain so you can't even think or act clearly.

We tennis players try so hard to play the perfect match, but we can always find something wrong with our game. It's like that in life, too. Making mistakes is normal. It's trying to correct them that really matters—staying in the solution. You have to acknowledge what you're doing wrong, then ask, "What do I need to do to correct it?" "What can I do better?" And then you figure it out and, hopefully, change it. That's an example of giving your best effort.

My childhood idol, Billie Jean King, planted some wise ideas in my head about the pursuit of excellence. When we worked together from 1989 to 1994, she encouraged me to be nicer to myself. I was so involved in being the best tennis player possible that I routinely gave myself a hard time whenever I fell short of my expectations. I'd kick myself for my mistakes and forget to take energy-boosting pleasure from what I did right. Billie Jean told me, "Sometimes you have to be satisfied. You try hard enough. Don't be so self-critical; don't be so hard on yourself."

So I took her advice to heart. I still set expectations for myself, but they involve doing my best rather than wanting to be the best. Sometimes I am still too hard on myself, but overall I am much better. These days, when reporters ask me how I will do in a certain tournament, I always tell them, "I have no expectations for doubles; I have no expectations for singles. The only expectation I ever have is to absolutely give my best effort, have a great time, enjoy myself, and hopefully put on a good show for the fans so that they'll enjoy it." It's amazing how your game picks up in the long run when you let up on yourself and give yourself permission to be less than perfect.

I like to keep a healthy perspective. Though I have a certain knack for a few things in life (I am a very good sleeper, for example, and my fruit-consuming skills are superb), I still have a lot of work to do on a lot of things, including my tennis game.

Sure, there's nothing wrong with wanting to build something special or extraordinary in any part of your life. The key, I think, is to strive to do things as well as you can rather than as perfectly as you can. If nothing else, you'll be rewarded with less stress. Whenever you notice that you're expecting too much of yourself, just tell yourself, "Let go of perfection." You'll feel calm, at peace, and more energized as you go after your goals.

So if you're ready to give your best effort, let's get started on the six steps to shape your self. The journey begins on the next page.

CHAPTER 2

STEP 1:
DEVELOP THE MENTALITY
OF AN ATHLETE

Defeat does not signal the end of a dream.

I'll never forget the day at Wimbledon in 2003 when my mixed doubles partner, Leander Paes, blacked out after hitting a smash, then clung to me for support as he crumpled to the ground. Obviously, something was very wrong. I didn't know it at the time, but he had temporarily lost his sight and all control of his balance. He had had a similar feeling once before, while warming up for another match, and we had all thought he was low on sugar (his eating habits left a little to be desired then). He recovered both times, but 2 months later, I realized what a miracle it really was that we won the Wimbledon mixed doubles title that year.

After Wimbledon, Leander's condition deteriorated. He complained of severe headaches and dizziness. Then, a week before the U.S. Open, he was rushed to a hospital and later admitted to the M. D. Anderson Cancer Center in Orlando. We canceled our plans to play in the U.S. Open that year. I did not want to compete without him. He was a true partner, and we had a special connection that couldn't be duplicated with anyone else. Our bond went far beyond just winning titles; being on the court with him was a treat every single time that we played.

At the hospital, doctors initially suspected a brain tumor. Understandably, Leander was terrified and shaken. All of a sudden, the titles, the riches, the halo of sports stardom seemed meaningless, trivial, and irrelevant. But even if the suspicion proved to be true, he vowed to fight until the very last, with the same determination, optimism, courage, and positive energy with which he battled his opponents on the court.

Tests revealed that the problem wasn't a brain tumor but a brain abscess caused by a parasite. An abscess is a bundle of immune cells and other material that forms when a part of the body is infected. The infection, which was treatable with antibiotics, could have been caused by eating contaminated food.

I called Leander about every other day when he was in the hospital. Imagine my surprise when I found out that he was already exercising and doing yoga every day. I was humbled, amazed, and inspired by his will to get back to the game of living. In a later interview about the illness, Leander said, "It taught me how fragile life can be."

How true!

He gave himself 6 months to fully recover because he didn't want to return to the court at 70 or even 80 percent of his former self, but rather at 100 percent. Recover he did, and return to the court he did. But Leander didn't stop there. He vowed to continue fighting the disease, both with money and with his celebrity, to create awareness about it in his homeland, India, where doctors suspect that 1 in 50 people has been exposed to the parasite.

The inspiration. The ability to overcome seemingly insurmountable challenges. The spirit to give their all. And much more. This is the mentality that athletes like Leander embody.

We played together again in 2004. At our first match, he bowed to me at one point after I hit a great shot, but I felt like bowing to him 10 times over. I was so lucky to be playing with him again.

Even though they have unique talents, gifts, and strengths, top athletes like Leander are regular people who face the same challenges, problems, and obstacles we all do. Yes, they're famous and on display, making them seem slightly different from the rest of humanity, but if you think about it, they embody what's possible within each of us. Top athletes dream big, they set high goals, they push themselves, they bounce back from defeat, they achieve. Even though you may not aspire to win Wimbledon or break a track-and-field record, applying the lessons of athletes can help you stay motivated to get in shape and achieve championship levels in every area of your life.

LIVE OUT YOUR DREAMS

I knew I wanted to be a great tennis player the night my father took me to the Sparta sports center in Prague, an arena where 10,000 people can watch a hockey game or a tennis match. The big attraction that night was Rod Laver, the redheaded left-hander from Australia. That was around the time he signed a big contract— for $100,000—to travel all over the world to play tennis. That was an unheard-of sum of money in those days, when you consider that my father brought in just $1,000 a year. It was the first time I realized that someone could actually make a living by playing tennis. I always knew I couldn't be a 9-to-5 worker, not ever. (In the Czech Republic, the workday was 7:00 to 3:00.) I just didn't know exactly how I was going to avoid it, though, until I saw Rod Laver touring and making good money as a professional tennis player.

That night, as we watched him, I was amazed by the power, agility, and drive he had. I saw him rocketing around the court, and I thought, "That's it, that's me, that's the player I want to be."

After seeing Laver play, I knew what world-class tennis was like. I began having dreams about winning on the famous Centre Court at Wimbledon. My father helped put that dream in my head because he believed I could be a great player. He would hit the ball to me for hours, telling me I would be a great champion. That dream was just as vivid in my dad's head as it was in mine. He'd tell people that I was going to be a Wimbledon champion someday, and I wasn't about to disagree with him. His dream for me kept mine alive.

After George Parma accepted me as a pupil, I'd take the commuter train into Prague to play tennis. There I was, this little pipsqueak of a 9-year-old, lugging all my equipment on the train. I would imagine people asking themselves, "Who is she?" And I would think to myself, "Someday, you'll know."

You see, I started telling myself when I was little that I'd be a great tennis player, and eventually, I started believing it. Later, I was able to live my dream. Once you start believing in yourself, anything is possible. Of course, I'm not suggesting that you can be an NBA basketball player if you're 4 feet 11 and haven't played much basketball. That's not believing in yourself; that's fantasy.

What I'm talking about, really, is visualization, a powerful tool that's used by athletes, performers, businesspeople, and others to achieve success. It's the process of creating detailed mental pictures of yourself achieving a goal or bettering your performance. With visualization, you form an image of what you want to do or become, whether it's losing weight, changing unhealthy behaviors, mastering a sport, winning a competition, improving your level of physical fitness, or overcoming an addiction. You imagine yourself doing it, and your brain then knows exactly what you want and finds a way to make it happen. For me, if I had already won a match in my mind, I had a better chance of winning it for real.

FOLLOWING THROUGH

- Begin to tell yourself something often—that you'll eat a more healthful diet, for example, or that you'll exercise or get in better shape. Before long, you'll start believing it. Once you start believing in yourself, your dreams take shape. The more you believe, the more you achieve.

- Focus on what you want to achieve, maybe for just a few minutes a day. What does it look like? What do you want to look like? How do you want to feel? How can you play it out in your mind? How do you see yourself living your dream? Create the vision in your head and make it vivid, down to the last detail.

- Adopt a clear vision of how you want your body to look someday. Imagine how your new body will look, how it will feel, how it will move. Be optimistic but realistic at the same time. Know what your body is capable of becoming rather than imagining yourself as a supermodel. Visualizing yourself in better shape can actually encourage your body to follow your mind's plan.

- Practice an action or situation in your head—athletes call this mental rehearsal—and do it over and over until you have it exactly right. The idea of mental rehearsal is to actually create the experience of success in your mind. Suppose you're going to a party, for example, where you'll be faced with lots of unhealthy food and drinks. Rehearse in your head how you'll control your cravings and resist temptation. Or maybe you're thinking about skipping your workout. Switch mental gears. Picture yourself at the gym, exercising and experiencing the positive feelings you get from your workout. Or perhaps you're set to compete in a sporting event. Visualize how to stand or move, how to swing the racquet or bat, how to run the field or court—whatever it takes to achieve a winning performance. When you regularly focus on a successful outcome, you increase your potential to make it reality.

- Give your dream a chance to come true. For example, I take skating lessons because I want to be the best ice hockey player I can be. Same with snowboarding, golf, or whatever. What you eat, what you drink, how you train, what you do with your body and your health—your whole life, really—is all in your power.

GIVE YOURSELF SOMETHING TO REACH FOR EVERY SINGLE DAY

Dreams don't automatically come true unless you set measurable, manageable goals to make them come true. Probably no one knows more about goal-setting than athletes. What they do is break everything down to daily goals in order to achieve more far-reaching goals. Each daily goal is like a rung on a ladder that helps an athlete climb, step by step, to the top. You can't just start at the top rung.

Another example: Ever notice how babies begin to take their first steps? They progress very, very slowly, from a crawl, to a reach, to a wobble, to a step. I think small, deliberate movements are the best and most permanent building blocks for a healthier lifestyle.

It has always been important to me to know that I can achieve my goals by making every day count. For example, one of my main goals was always to be number one at the end of each year. So I'd break that objective down into smaller ones: What will help me perform the best today for what I need to do? What do I need to change? What do I need to eat? What do I need to drink? When do I need to eat? How much sleep do I need? If you do this, the trek to your goal isn't as long, and the objective isn't as overwhelming. Everything you do today impacts the next day as well as the future.

It just makes sense that if you concentrate on achieving small, doable, and manageable goals each day—and then you do the same thing again tomorrow, and the next day, and the next—you set yourself up for success.

The choices you make and the actions you take today will add up. If you focus on what you need to do today, achieving your bigger goals, like losing 20 pounds or getting fit enough to compete in a marathon, will be easier. If you do your best today, tomorrow will take care of itself.

FOLLOWING THROUGH

- Set small daily goals. They are easier to reach, and when you accomplish them, you'll have a sense of success and the forward momentum it brings. When you get up in the morning, you might choose one or two goals for the day, such as eating more fruits and vegetables, not eating so many sugary or fatty foods, cutting out sodas, drinking more water, going to an exercise class, or practicing some form of stress management to avoid emotional overeating. When you feel empowered by achieving daily goals, you're more likely to keep climbing that ladder—and get to the top of your game, whatever that is.
- Make sure your goals are measurable, such as time, distance, or quantity. When I run a mile on the track, for example, I time myself because I have a specific goal for how fast I want to run. If I previously did a 7:45 mile, I want to do a 7:35 one the next time. I like to be able to measure what I do because I need to see progress to keep myself going. Wearing a heart rate monitor or a pedometer to count

steps can help you measure progress, too. Diet-wise, keeping track of what and how much you eat is a way to help you stay the course and establish healthier eating habits.
- Set flexible goals. Your goals need to be flexible enough to accommodate the unexpected. Life is always changing. If your goal is to run in a certain race, and you are injured, you may have to modify that goal, compete in a different event, or postpone running until you're healed. You don't give up on your plans; you adjust.
- Acknowledge all of your efforts. If you've given your goals your all, putting your heart into them, don't beat yourself up if you don't quite make it. Whenever people ask me how many Wimbledons I've won, I say, "Nine; could've been 10, but I'm not complaining." Sure, I remember the one that got away, but rather than express regret, I am thankful for every accomplishment. The key is to have the same attitude toward goal-setting. If you do, you'll move through your life with far greater success.

PUT IT IN WRITING

Katharine Hepburn used to tell me, "Keep notes. Keep track of what you're doing." Back then, 20 years ago, I couldn't be bothered. I didn't pay enough attention. I thought I'd remember the important things. But you don't.

On her advice, though, I finally began a journal in the 1980s. I wanted to track my results, monitor my progress, jot down notes about my performance, and zero in on areas that needed improvement.

I wrote in it sporadically until 1989, when Billie Jean King, who was helping me at the time, and Craig Kardon, my full-time coach, urged me to write down everything that was happening—at practice, during workouts, on the tennis court, and with my body. You see, there was a very important, very big goal looming—the opportunity to win Wimbledon for the ninth time. No one had ever won nine Wimbledons, and I wanted to be the first. Not surprisingly, the media had largely written me off, thinking I didn't have a chance.

July 7, 1990, was a day I'll remember all my life. My opponent was Zina Garrison, to whom I had lost only once in 27 matches. I'll admit it, I was nervous, but I was feeling so good, so confident.

In what would be the last point, I watched Zina hit a passing shot way long. My hands flew into the air, and my knees sank into the lush turf. I had won my ninth Wimbledon and broken the record held for 52 years by Helen Wills Moody, the American who was the dominant woman player in the 1920s and 1930s.

What part journaling played in my victory—coincidence or connection—I don't really know for sure. All I can say is that when I got serious about journaling, I won that Wimbledon. I also know that writing everything down, as Billie Jean advised me to do, helped me absorb the technical and emotional improvements I had to make to my game if I were ever to win Wimbledon again.

Since then, I've been pretty religious about making tennis-related entries in my journal. Whenever I learn something new, I write it down. When I need to work on something—

like lowering the toss on my serve, jumping more into the court, or anything technical or tactical that I've been working on—I write it down. When one of my opponents has a tendency to do something at a particular time in a match, I write that down, too, so that when I play that person again, I can go back to that entry and recall it. Before a match, I always review my tennis entries. This has helped me outthink my opponents. It helps me set up a strategy, and then the match unfolds as I predicted it would.

Beyond its application to tennis, I've also found that journaling can be a powerful tool for self-discovery, to wake up that part of you under the surface that needs to come out in the light—which is why I write notes to help sort through and express my feelings. When you write about your emotions, the lows as well as the highs, you can deal with them much better. There's a part of me, for example, that is afraid of failure, of not living up to other people's expectations or my own. Writing about it takes the power away from the fear, and I feel much more confident. We don't acknowledge many of our fears, preferring instead to adopt the ostrich's head-in-the-sand mentality. But if you confront what's bothering you by putting your thoughts down on paper, you can do something about it. You may even realize that the problem is much smaller than you originally thought.

Keeping a journal of what's going on in your life is a good way to help you distill what's important and what's not—in the same way that going on a camping trip teaches you exactly what you need so that next time, you don't take more than what is absolutely essential. For example, if you write about your eating habits, you may discover that you're eating too much of what you don't need and not enough of what you do need.

Journaling keeps you mindful of what you're doing, mindful of what works, and mindful of what doesn't work. That way, you can eliminate what doesn't work so you won't make the same mistakes over and over again. The fewer mistakes you make twice, the easier life is.

Using your journal, you can clarify your goals, whatever they are—where you'd like to see yourself physically, emotionally, intellectually, and professionally. I journal even the mundane, like my to-do lists.

You can also write about what you're grateful for, as a way to count your blessings. The reason this is so powerful is that it keeps you focused on the better parts of what you have.

Here's a personal example: Growing up in the Czech Republic made me appreciate everything I have. I'm still amazed that I can go to a grocery store and buy anything I want without having to wait in line. Now there are more modern grocery stores there, but as a young kid, I'd have to go to buy bread and milk and butter every other day because we didn't have a refrigerator, and there was always a line. Anybody who complains about life should go to a place like Kenya, as I did several years ago. It will give them a different perspective. The women have to carry water and huge piles of firewood a couple of miles every day just to cook their meals. Drinking water is a precious commodity there, and most households have no electricity. Here, we take all those things for granted. That made such an impression on me

that I always turn off the water when I'm brushing my teeth. These are the kinds of things I write about in my journal—the deeper appreciation for what I have and how easy my life really is. Once you make journaling a regular part of your life, I think you will like how good it can make you feel.

FOLLOWING THROUGH

- Start the journaling process by buying a book that is pleasing to you. My journal is a leather-bound book, but a journal doesn't have to be fancy. A simple spiral notebook may be all you need. Its pages can be lined or unlined, in case you want to draw in it.
- Be creative. Consider writing your entries in prose, poetry, diary, or letter form. The key is to personalize your journal for your life and make it meaningful.
- Write about anything of significance to you. Your journal entries can be to-do notes, events in your life, goals you've set and met, decisions you've made, problems that need resolution, emotions you're dealing with, insights you've picked up in life, or quotes you want to remember.
- Add entries whenever you feel the urge to pick up your journal and write. Or set aside a specific time to write each day if you can. If time is a problem, at least try to manage a weekly journaling session.
- Keep your entries concrete. That is, include enough factual material so that when you go back and read it, you will know what you've written about and can properly reflect on it.
- Reread your journal periodically. This will help you stay focused, remind you of the

goals you've set, and let you see how far you've come toward accomplishing them.

FOCUS ON STAYING IN THE MOMENT

Chris Evert once told me about a time when she was playing in the finals at a major tournament back in the seventies, and she took her mind off the match for a split second and lost the point. What happened was that she saw her former fiancé, Jimmy Connors, in the stands with his new girlfriend. It rattled her since she and Jimmy, once dubbed the "Lovebird Double," had recently called off their engagement, and she was still in love with him. She lost focus, and her game momentarily fell apart.

More recently, tennis superstar Venus Williams dropped in the rankings. The reason, according to some, was the fact that she started an interior design business. I can't say for sure that was the reason; all I know is that tennis requires tremendous focus and a huge amount of mental discipline. If I were coaching Venus, I wouldn't want her to be thinking about color palettes for houses; I would want her focused on tennis. It's hard for me to believe that you can compete on that level and have your mind elsewhere. If Michael Jordan had decided to become an architect at the height of his career with the Chicago Bulls, I can't believe that would have been considered a good career move. But, as they say, to each his own.

It's not uncommon for athletes to lose focus. If you're playing tennis and something distracts you, you end up not totally concentrating on what you need to accomplish. You miss an easy

shot, so you scream or shake your head while your opponent scores the next point. You're still shaking your head when you miss the next point. Then you're *still* shaking your head because you missed two points ago, and now you're totally not thinking about what you need to do next. Pretty soon, that one missed point has cost you three games! It has happened to me more times than I care to remember. One time, right in the middle of a match at Wimbledon, I watched a small plane circling overhead, trailing a banner that said "Use the Postal Code." I wondered why anybody would pay tax money to hire a plane to advertise that message, and then I started thinking about all the letters I owed people and tried to remember their ZIP codes. While my mind was wandering, my opponent won a few games in the second set. I needed to refocus and get my act together.

How do I regain focus when I've gotten out of the flow? What helps me most of all is identifying beforehand what will typically distract me, then deliberately avoiding it. In tennis, I used to find it hard to concentrate when an opponent was also my friend. For instance, I would make a point not to catch my friend Pam Shriver's eye in the locker room (in tennis, opponents don't have separate dressing rooms) before we played each other in singles. I knew if she arched those eyebrows of hers, she'd have me laughing, and I wouldn't be able to totally concentrate on my match.

There was also a time when listening to the highlights of a tournament on television the night before an important match disrupted my peace of mind, especially if something controversial was aired. The mute button came in handy at that point.

Losing focus happens in life just as it does in athletics. When you have so much else on your mind, you're distracted from what you need to be doing now. That's why it's so important to stay in the moment. Take your time, do everything you can to take care of yourself, enjoy the process, and before you know it, you will have lost the weight, kicked the bad habit, firmed up your body, or achieved whatever else it is you set out to do.

Where people go astray, however, is that they get too focused on, and sometimes obsessed with, the end result. They worry about how many pounds they've lost this week or that week. If their weight loss doesn't meet their expectations, they get discouraged and depressed. You can't predict how much weight you'll lose from week to week anyway, because it takes a while for the body to adjust to what's going on, and the results may not be immediate. You might lose 5 pounds the first week and none the next, even if you've been true to your diet. Plus, thinking about the end result—how you need to lose 50 or 100 pounds—can be overwhelming, and that can make you want to give up. You need to break it down—concentrate on what you need to do *today* to reach that goal—then just continue to take it a day at a time. Besides, if you get obsessed about losing weight, it probably won't happen because you are worrying too much. Why? Because chronic stress and worry, like lack of sleep, can elevate levels of cortisol, a fat-producing hormone. Worry is always self-defeating, even when it comes to the size of your waistline.

I believe that if you can stay focused on the present, enjoying each day and celebrating that day's success, you'll move confidently toward attaining your greater goals. It's all about staying mindful of the present moment instead of mentally fast-forwarding to a future that hasn't arrived yet.

FOLLOWING THROUGH

- Concentrate on concentrating. How often have you sat at your desk at work and pondered what you're going to make for dinner? Or worried over last night's quarrel with your partner while making a presentation or participating in an important meeting? Too often, we drift away from what's happening to us right now to fret over the past or future. As a result, our attention is scattered, and we don't do a good job with either the task at hand or the one that's distracting us. I believe that your mind can be productive in only one place—the past, the present, or the future. You have to make a decision: Do you want to stay distracted, or do you want to think about what you're doing now? Of course your mind is going to wander. When it does, be aware that your thoughts are drifting and quickly bring them back to the now, to the moment. By living in the moment, we can make better choices and live more productive lives.

- Make lists. Getting organized by making lists of what you need to do is one of the best ways to maintain—and regain—focus. It's always hectic around my house when I'm headed out of town for some tournaments, for example, and it's easy to forget what needs to be done. I make two lists—one for me and one for my assistant. Once I write everything down, I take care of it. Then I can say, "Okay, I can let go of that." This frees me to concentrate on other things that need to be done.

- Focus on your short-term, immediate goals. People tell me all the time that their minds roam when they're training or working out in the gym. My advice? Make a mental list of what you want to accomplish during a workout or training session; these are short-term goals. Do you want to run for a full 60 minutes? Do you want to up your weight on biceps curls? Do you want to do both strength training and aerobics in a single workout? Do you want to keep up with your training partner? Having immediate goals like these, and knowing them beforehand, helps keep your mind where it should be—on your workout.

- Relax. Often, just some simple relaxation moves will sharpen your focusing skills. When you feel like you're zoning out, take three or more slow breaths. Concentrate on your breathing and the position of your body and begin to visualize how your body is slimming down and getting stronger. This form of meditation will pull your mind back to where it needs to be.

HAVE THE WILL TO PREPARE

One of my favorite quotes is from Joe Paterno, the great football coach from Penn State. He said, "The will to win is important, but the will to prepare is vital." Top athletes know this, and they're willing to put in the time to really work at their sport. In tennis, for example, it's not an accident when you hit a great shot, because you've done it in practice. You've put in the work. Every great shot you hit, you've already hit a bunch of times in practice.

It's like getting ready for an exam. You have to study all the books, all your notes, all your material. You can't just show up for the exam and hope it includes the right questions. Your preparation has to be all-encompassing.

I'll give you some personal examples. To this day, if I play a lousy match, I head right to the practice court to hit. It isn't always after a loss, either; it may be after a win, when I still want to work on something. If I win a match but stink up the joint, I get out to a practice court and get it figured out before the next match. You want to be ready for the next time, whenever that is. And if it's tomorrow, then you'd better get it right tonight.

Last year in India, my coach and I realized that for me to really see the ball and be ready, I need to literally play with the ball before I go on the court. For about 20 minutes, I throw it up against the wall, dribble it, toss it up, and catch it. The idea is to get my eyes tuned in to the ball. When I was younger, there was no need to do this, since my eyes and reflexes were sharper. But now that I'm older, I have to keep reinforcing the sensation even more—seeing the ball and getting mentally attuned to it. This exercise is terrific preparation. It gets me ready from the first point, and that's as it should be.

You can extend this idea of preparation to yourself and use it to help every aspect of your life. To be prepared for a healthy, productive lifestyle is to live one.

FOLLOWING THROUGH

- Go grocery shopping with a list of healthy foods (and stick to it so you don't buy unhealthy impulse items!).
- Trim your kitchen as you trim yourself. Clear away unhealthy foods and restock your kitchen with healthy choices only.
- Plan your meals day by day or week by week. Stick to your plan. Using a daily or weekly meal planner is a huge help.
- Cut up veggies or prepare other healthy snacks the night before work.
- Be familiar with restaurant menus so you can go to places that serve healthy food.
- Eat before you go to a party so you won't overindulge when you get there.
- Pack your gym bag the night before a workout day and have it ready to go.

PUSH YOURSELF TO GREATER HEIGHTS

Every champion is driven by a competitive urge to win. Though you don't necessarily have to beat other people on the playing field, a very powerful motivator is to be competitive with yourself. When I was little, for example, I would run around the garden to see how fast I could go. Nobody was watching me, nobody knew— but me. Even today, I enjoy competing against myself to see how well I can play and if I can play better than I did the last time. When I play ice hockey with the Mother Puckers in Aspen, I know that there are better players and better skaters on the team than me. I'll never be as good as they are, but I want to be as good as *I* can be.

Having this attitude is one of the key reasons I have been able to develop as an athlete. I'm sure if you give it a try, it will work for you, too.

You have absolute control over your personal level of fitness. If you push yourself to new heights, stay competitive with yourself, and give it your best shot, then chances are, you're going to look and feel great. You'll be strong and fit. And you'll learn to be proud of yourself because you've changed for the better.

FOLLOWING THROUGH

- Push yourself nutritionally by working more variety into your meals. Expand your food choices by trying some exotic new fruit, vegetable, or other food.
- Break your own records. For example, challenge yourself to run that mile a little faster each time you work out, exercise five times a week instead of three, or increase the distance you walk on the treadmill.
- If you truly enjoy competition, why not enter a race, such as a 5-K or a 10-K, or start training for a marathon? Whether you win or lose, the main thing is that you have stretched yourself—by improving your coordination and strength, by sharpening your physical and mental skills, and by experiencing the fun and teamwork. Remember, it's not the score that counts, or whether you brought home a trophy. If you're in there just to win, that moment goes by very quickly. So what if you're happy for 5 minutes? The world doesn't really care. It's what's inside you that matters. It's about the desire to do the best you can, whatever that is, every day you get out of bed. It's about enjoying the process,

not the end result. When you do that, you're already a winner.

LEARN TO BOUNCE BACK

One of the toughest things athletes face is training for their sport, then competing and not winning or even getting close. Every athlete experiences this; none of us has a never-ending winning streak.

One of the lowest points in my career occurred during 1976, a year after I defected to the United States. What I thought was going to be easy—moving to America and playing on tour—was anything but. I was not yet 20, very much on my own, and very alone—alone in my hotel room, alone in airplanes. I was irritable, sad, and lonely, with few friends and no place to call home.

I stayed constantly on the go. That year, I was playing for the Cleveland Nets, one of the teams with World Team Tennis, a new league at the time. Then I played Wimbledon, where I lost to Chris Evert but got my first Wimbledon title by winning doubles with her. Afterward, I was back on the plane for a Nets match in San Francisco. I played something like 12 matches in 14 days and continued in pretty much the same vein for the rest of July and August. That gave me 2 weeks to rest and get ready for the U.S. Open that year—hardly enough time. If you don't put in enough practice, it catches up with you. I was so tired after that long run that I actually took the 2 weeks off and hit the ball only on Saturday and Sunday before the Open.

Playing against Janet Newberry, I won the first set, 6–1. But then I fell apart, doing everything wrong, lunging at the ball, and the match started getting away from me. Janet won the next two sets, and I was out. I walked off the court just sobbing, with tears rolling down my face. For the first and only time in my career, I ducked the press because I was so miserable. It wasn't nice, the way I acted. I just didn't have any control over myself at the time.

I still consider that loss the worst of my career, at least in the way I responded to it on and off the court. So much was expected of me, so much happened to me that year, that I felt like the whole world was crashing in on me. It was hard for me to adjust to losing because I had come along so fast that I didn't know what it was like to struggle. I just knew it felt like the world was going to end.

I was like a ship without its anchor, adrift and lost, and what I needed most of all was an anchor. I had always had my home in the Czech Republic to go back to, but not anymore. So I did what made sense to me at the time. Soon after my loss to Newberry, I went to Dallas and bought a house. I knew the city. I had friends there, so it made sense to settle in. Right away, I felt more at home. My way of bouncing back was to get anchored.

There have been other times in my life when I didn't feel right about my game, times when I couldn't hit the wide side of a barn if my life depended on it. To get back in gear again, I knew I had to train harder, make adjustments, and refine my game so I could come back stronger and better than ever.

You know what I'm talking about if you've ever fallen short of your health goals by slipping up on your diet, getting lazy exercise-wise, or not following your doctor's orders. These things happen; you can count on it. You have to be prepared to take some nicks along the way.

The only way you can fail at building a healthy lifestyle is if you give up. As long as you pick yourself up after a setback and get back into the game as top athletes do, you have a great chance to succeed.

FOLLOWING THROUGH

- Rethink your goals. Maybe your original goals were too lofty or unrealistic. You can motivate yourself a lot more, and prevent possible setbacks, by focusing on goals that are more attainable, especially over the short term.
- Learn from your experience. Take something positive from it. What lessons can you take away? That you have trouble eating healthy at restaurants or parties? That you don't like a certain type of workout? Don't beat yourself up over it. Learn from it, gather information to help you succeed, and move on. You've got to. Whatever your slipup was, determine what you can do to prevent it from happening again. That's what great athletes do: They convert setbacks into strengths. In other words, they know how to bounce back.
- Remember how far you have come. Take note of how much strength you've gained, the fat you've lost, how much better you look in your clothes; appreciate your newfound energy. Noting your progress will help reinforce your commitment to a healthy lifestyle.
- Keep your sense of humor. Look for an amusing aspect in everything, even your setbacks.

DON'T SNOOZE THROUGH LIFE'S WAKE-UP CALLS

As I close this chapter, I'd like to talk to you about wake-up calls—those critical moments that give you the opportunity to transform your life in positive ways. If you grab hold of those opportunities, you can become better than you have ever been—healthier, stronger, leaner, happier, more successful—and stay that way for the rest of your life.

Throughout my tennis career, it's clear that I've had lots of wake-up calls, usually in the form of my performance. When it's not that great, that tells me that I need to do something different or something better if I'm to play well that year. Good athletes listen to those wake-up calls, whether they come in the form of an injury, not making the cut, a losing streak, a losing season, or other signs that things have to be different. They know that these signs are catalysts for change and are wise enough to learn from them.

As far as some wake-up calls go, however, some athletes have a habit of hitting the snooze button and going back to sleep. They think they're bulletproof. They believe they can drive drunk, jam steroid-filled needles into their buttocks, take sexual risks, or get in trouble with the law without any consequences whatsoever. It's sad, really sad.

Life continually presents us with wake-up calls regarding our health. What happened to my friend Paul is a good example. A resident of

New York City, Paul is a really unusual fellow whom I met early in my career. When I was introduced to him, he asked me to call him not Paul but "Wally." I couldn't make the leap from Paul to Wally, so I asked, "Why Wally?" He answered, "Look at me! If I were an animal, what kind of animal would I look like?"

At first I thought he was kidding me, but then I looked at him closely: pure white hair slicked back and falling to his shoulders and a bright red, round face with a full mustache stretching beyond his chin. As he stood in front of me in a deliberately animated pose, I began to laugh out loud. He had a very long, broad frame with a rather round midsection. Yes, with his exaggerated pose, even through a child's eyes, he colorfully resembled a walrus, albeit a very cute baby one.

Paul is a sweet man, extremely funny, and a person who truly puts the capital L in life. I remember once running into him on the streets of New York during the Christmas season. He was dressed in a Santa Claus suit, and when he saw me, he ran up to me, yelling, "Hey, little girl, what kind of racquet are you in?" I didn't recognize him at first, until he struck his familiar walrus pose.

During my off-season, we often had meals together. The first time I had dinner with him, he said that since he was on a diet, he would like to look at the menu of each restaurant before we decided on one. After checking about 20 restaurants, he suggested one of his favorites, a deli. I was starving, so I agreed. We sat down, talked a bit, and then ordered. I went first, ordering blintzes. Paul then placed his order: a bowl of split pea soup, a Greek salad with chicken, brisket with extra gravy on the potatoes, and pecan pie with vanilla ice cream and whipped topping for dessert.

Now, that didn't sound like any diet I was aware of, so I asked, "Hey, Paul, going off the diet for tonight?"

"Nope," he said. "Haven't finished my order. I'll have a Tab." Ordering a diet cola was his idea of being on a diet.

Throughout a usual day, he ate meals similar to the one I witnessed, always with a Tab. This way of "dieting" went on for many years, until one very stressful day when, during a heated discussion at work, his nose started bleeding profusely. He became so faint that he was rushed to the nearest hospital, where he was diagnosed with life-threatening hypertension. Upon release, he was given a rather lengthy "strict diet"—a real one—that was started during his hospital stay. This drastic change from his usual diet to the real deal altered his eating habits forever. Wake-up calls don't get much louder.

Today, he is a very healthy middle-aged grandfather, looking forward to walking his youngest daughter down the aisle at her upcoming wedding. During one of our more recent dinners in New York, he made a toast to himself, "for kicking the knucklehead in me to the curb and taking charge of my health so that I could enjoy this day with my wife, children, grandchildren, and great friends." To this day, he still reflects on how it took a traumatic event to change his life. He often comments on how many of his associates over the years have had similar experiences. Some are still living, while others never had a chance to change.

What makes people like Paul have the resolve to change, while so many other people live with shoulda, woulda, coulda? They've had wake-up calls, and when the calls came, they answered.

How about you? Do you see those extra pounds or the last bad health report as a serious sign that your life has to change? I hope you'll take your wake-up calls to heart, questioning every area of your health, and live deliberately so you get the most out of your life.

The best athletes are students of their game. They put in their mental work as much as their physical work. It's what propels them to the top. When you have the right mentality, with your dreams and goals clearly in mind, with the mental toughness it takes to focus, bounce back, and listen to wake-up calls, everything you want for yourself will begin to materialize—and that's exciting.

There's one more element you need to set your course toward real change: supportive relationships that encourage your success. In order to succeed, you need people on your "team" who will pull for you, prop you up when you've fallen down, and push you forward when you've lost your momentum. Keep turning the pages, and you'll find out how to get those people on your team.

CHAPTER 3

STEP 2:
BUILD YOUR
SUPPORT TEAM

The right people can inspire you to do the right things.

In the Czech Republic, we have a proverb: "Do not protect yourself by a fence, but rather by your friends." My life in many ways has been a reflection of that proverb, and I think making a commitment to change your lifestyle must involve having a support system of friends and family around you.

All the time I was growing up, I had a lot of friends. I still do—friends who know me but love me, support me, encourage me, and watch out for me anyway! I can count on them, no matter what the circumstance.

When we were kids, my friends and I were always playing something—hopscotch, pitching pennies, cowboys and Indians, or sports like ice hockey and soccer. By the time I was 10, however, tennis had separated me from the other kids in Revnice, my hometown. One or two days a week, I'd hustle out of school and catch the train into Prague for tennis practice. By the time I got home, I barely had enough time to do my homework before I fell asleep. This cut out a lot of time for friendships that the other kids had.

As I was becoming a tennis player, my family was my main support system—my "team"—for helping me meet my goals. I spent hundreds of hours learning the game of tennis with my father and mother at the Revnice tennis club. Both my parents had such a zest for the sport that I know it was contagious. While they were playing club matches, I'd practice for hours, just hitting against the wall. I remember the time my father took me to play tennis on a real court and taught me how to hit a forehand. I was probably about 7 years old at the time. The moment I stepped onto that crunchy red clay, felt the grit under my sneakers, felt the joy of smacking a ball over the net, I knew I was in the right place.

Overall, in that time of a crumbling and communist Czech economy, our family had a good life compared to most other people. We had our own house, and my father had a good job as an economist in a factory. My mother went to work, too, yet she never stopped caring for me and my younger sister, Jana, in every detail. Mom has always been very sweet, very giving, very maternal. As for my father, he told me all about tennis. He taught me to play aggressively. He told me to rush the net, put it past opponents, take a chance, invent shots. It was his advice, his energy, his enthusiasm, that gave me my chance in tennis.

Though he was the disciplinarian in the house, my father had a fun, playful streak, and he was always joking with us. When I was about 7, I remember him taking me swimming in the Berounka River near our house and throwing me in, then picking me up. When it came to swimming, my athletic ability usually failed me; I just wasn't a good swimmer as a kid. One time, he threw me in a different place where there was a big hole in the bottom of the river. I disappeared underneath the water and almost drowned. My dad dived in after me, but he couldn't find me because the river

was so silty that it was hard to see anything. He came back up for air, and the second time he went under, he grabbed me. I came up sputtering. We were just playing around, and the next thing you know, it was a life-threatening situation.

That may be an extreme example, but it illustrates some things your support system does for you—rescues you if you need it, gives you strength when you're weak, cares for you, helps you, and keeps you out of harm's way, whatever that may be. Above all, both my parents gave me the greatest gift any child could receive— they believed in me.

TEAM NAVRATILOVA

When I first came to the States in the seventies, I was without a coach for about 7 years, so I was pretty much on my own. I didn't have much support in that regard, and I didn't even know to ask for help. It's hard to get motivated day in and day out by yourself. How could I fix my strokes if there was no one watching me? I know I could have won more with the guidance of a coach, but I did the best I could.

Gradually, though, people began to notice me, and friendships started to spring up with important tennis people. But at that point, I didn't really have a formal support system. That all changed in 1981.

That was the year I had my midlife crisis— and I was only 26! I believed I was already "over the hill" athletically. I was losing matches because I was too tired and too slow to run for the ball, and there was no reason for that to happen. One thing you can control in life is the shape you're in. If you run for the ball and you miss it—well, okay, at least you've had a chance to miss it. But if you can't even get there because you're too tired to run, or you're not fast enough because you're in poor shape—there's no excuse for that.

It was Nancy Lieberman who bluntly told me at that point in my life, "Martina, you're wasting your talent!" She was right. If I did win a match, it was because I was getting by on sheer talent only. I was not playing up to my potential. Time was running out; 30—that age when athletes are supposed to retire—was right around the corner. I needed to get my act together.

At this point, I had already won two Wimbledons—and I had worked hard, no question about that. But there was another level I could take it to. I decided to go for it.

First, I had to get in much better physical shape, which involved a lot of help from Nancy. Then I hired a coach: Dr. Renee Richards, who started helping me during the U.S. Open that year. And nutritionist Robert Haas came around at about the same time, redesigning my diet. There was a convergence of talent that really changed my career and my life. Nancy used to call it Team Navratilova. The team helped me get started and eventually reach my potential as a tennis player. Getting there was (and still is) a work in progress.

Probably one of the newest things in this mix was the workout. It was at that time a pretty sophisticated training program, and very specific to tennis. I did drills for footwork and positioning, drills for balance, drills for reaction time, and drills to develop parts of the body that were used by tennis players. I worked with Lynn Conkwright, a former champion bodybuilder, who designed a daily weight-training program for me.

The hard work and the teamwork paid off, taking me to a new level of strength, endurance, and quickness that ultimately led to winning most of my Grand Slam titles between 1982 and 1987. Even though I have weighed pretty much the same since 1977—between 143 and 150 pounds—it was only in 1981 that I got in great shape physically, and I have been able to stay that way since. Sure, I've had a few hiccups in controlling my weight, but I've managed to keep it within a healthy range.

THE SUPPORTIVE SPIRIT OF TEAMWORK

On the tennis tour, most of the women have always been supportive of each other, and we need that. Everybody does. Chris Evert and others have consoled me after a loss, and I've done the same for them. We women were always good at getting along. We spent a lot of time with each other, and I guess that's part of it, but we also seem to have an instinct for nurturing within us. We want to get along with people, smooth things over. Sure, we're competitive, but we're subtle about it. Some of my best friends off the court have also been my rivals on the court.

Chris, of course, is the best-known example of what I'm talking about. Most people who follow sports like to think that ours was one of the greatest rivalries in the history of sports. All I know is that there has never been another rivalry like the Chris and Martina show, and I don't think there ever will be. For 15 straight years, from March 1973 to November 1988, we battled each other 80 times, a record in individual-sports history. We played 60 finals and 22 times in Grand Slam tournaments (14 finals), and our overall score was 43–37 in my favor. During that time, we were like chocolate-or-vanilla, jazz-or-classical—two champions with opposing styles and temperaments. I was the aggressive net rusher and Chris the patient baseliner, and we were competing for limited space at the top of women's tennis.

Chris has often said, "We brought out the best in each other." That is so true. I remember when she showed up on the tour in 1984 in better shape than I had ever seen her. She had been working with weights and using some of the other conditioning techniques I had been using, and she was strong. Chris had previously said that she would rather lose a point than fall to the ground trying to make one, but after she had lost many times in a row to me, she got serious about her conditioning program. Likewise, I had to keep fine-tuning my game to keep up with Chris's precision passing shots. We kept raising the level of our games as we both improved.

We have always been great friends too, taking pride in being fair with each other. Many, many years ago, I pleaded with Chris, "Please change racquets. Use a metal one instead of a wooden one. You won't believe the difference. You will hit the ball harder, and you will play better."

I wanted to help her be a better player. I didn't want to beat her because I had a better racquet. I wanted to level the playing field so we both had the same opportunity. Once you do that, you can see who is the better player. Fairness has always been the main thing to me. I think the history that Chris and I have shared is a great example of friends and rivals pushing each other to achieve greater goals and supporting each other off the court.

Today, one of the reasons I'm still playing doubles—besides the fact that I can—is that I love teaming up with someone else. As the old saying goes, there is no "I" in "team." My doubles game is as important as my singles game always was. It's not just Navratilova; it's Navratilova and my partner—whomever I may be paired with at the time. My partner has carried me sometimes, and I've carried my partner sometimes, but we've mainly been a team.

I am a firm believer in strength in numbers. No athlete, whether in a team sport or an individual sport like tennis, reaches the top without support. Chris had a Team Evert long before I had a support system of my own. Her father, Jimmy, who was her first coach and who reinforced her love for tennis, didn't go on the road very often, but her mother, Collette, was often there, as were her sister Jeanne, a tour player herself, and a number of their friends. Chris didn't know what it was like to be alone on tour.

Tiger Woods, arguably the best golfer in the world, has on his team a personal trainer, a physical therapist, and a golf instructor who works with him in intensive, daylong practice sessions prior to major tournaments. Tiger never quits learning or bettering his game. He soaks up information like a sponge. That's why he's the best.

The often-controversial baseball player

Barry Bonds, an unprecedented four-time MVP, is an example of an athlete who plays on a team but has his own support crew: a nutritionist, a chef, and three trainers. His team has been called the best support system in the history of baseball by *Baseball Digest*.

Surrounding myself with family, friends, teammates, coaches, trainers, and other advisors has helped me become a tennis champion and play the best tennis any woman has ever played—which I think I have done for a good part of my career.

You don't have to be an elite athlete, though, to build a support system. Anyone who wants to improve their health habits and get in better shape, physically and mentally, would do well to get support from friends, family, and others. Having a support system increases your motivation, so you try harder and even get in shape faster. No matter what your fitness level or goals, support can take you to the next level. It's the extra boost that can keep you going when you feel like giving up. It can restore your flow when you're at a low ebb. And it can make the difference between success and failure. I guess the best thing about a support system is that you always have people on your side.

GRAVITATE TOWARD PEOPLE WHO ARE GOOD FOR YOU

When you are ready to make changes in your life, gather the support from around you. The right people won't let you cheat on your diet or ignore your workouts. I remember Nancy Lieberman asking me, "When are you going out to practice?" I would tell her that I didn't

necessarily practice every day, and when I did practice, I usually didn't go for more than an hour. She'd insist that I work harder, giving it more than I ever had. Or she'd say, "Martina, don't you think we ought to go to the gym?" She was really good at prodding me to get in shape at a time when I needed it. Because I respected her as an athlete and as a person, I paid attention to what she said. She had credibility, and that's something important you want in a support system. With Nancy keeping watch over me and being my friend, I had the support to start training harder than I ever had in the past.

Of course, you want to be around positive people who will help you get to a goal or who make you feel good about being around them, whether it's a physical feel-good, an emotional feel-good, or a stimulating mental feel-good. How do you know if somebody will be a positive influence on you? You can tell a lot about people by the way they act and interact—how they carry themselves, how they dress, and whether they look you in the eye during conversations. How do they treat servers in restaurants? Do they deal with them as human beings or treat them as if they're subservient? Are they compassionate? Are they respectful of other people? Can they admit their mistakes?

Pay attention to the signals people send. You can learn a lot by observing. Here's a case in point: After she retired, Chris Evert told me, "I always knew if you were going to play well, depending on how you acted in the locker room."

"What are you talking about?" I said, surprised.

She said, "Well, if you were talking a lot, I

knew you were confident. And if you were quiet, I knew you were nervous."

I laughed. "Oh, I had no idea. Thanks for telling me now!"

Chris is tuned in to people. She has great powers of observation. That's what you need if you are to fill your life with people who are positive.

Positive people are dependable, they make fitness fun, and they are as committed to good health as you are. They bring upbeat, inspiring energy to your efforts.

FOLLOWING THROUGH

- As it did for Nancy and me, it helps if you and your friends or family share the same value system when it comes to nutrition, exercise, and health in general.
- Work out or train with people who are at your level or a little bit better and who are on the same page with you health-wise, so you can try to get better in every way. I always try to play tennis with people who are a little better than I am because they can push me further.
- If you're in a relationship, try exercising with your partner as a way to spend quality time together, not to mention turning a routine workout into an exciting, fun, and even sensual experience.
- Participate in a sports group, such as a biking club, tennis or racquetball league, or walking club. All of these have built-in support systems made possible by their group settings.
- Find a workout buddy.
- Within your support system, have everyone promise to encourage each other with uplifting words at least once a day. Having someone say "I am proud of you" can inspire you to stay the course.

LEARN TO DEAL WITH NEGATIVE PEOPLE

I once had a group of friends who wanted to order a bottle of wine every time we went out. I'd take a little sip, and they'd polish off the rest—then debate whether to order another bottle. They were drinking a lot and urging me to do the same, and I wouldn't. I just didn't like being with people like that. When people try to sabotage me, I just don't hang out with them; I'd rather be alone. You don't want to go out to dinner and have people make you feel bad because you won't eat french fries or have an alcoholic drink.

One woman told me that whenever she wanted to stay faithful to her diet, she had to avoid being with her friends because they completely invalidated her efforts by picking the most diet-unfriendly places to meet and have dinner. On one particular occasion, she suggested a restaurant where the cuisine fit her diet choices. The response from her friends was so unsupportive and so counterproductive to her efforts that she just stopped going out with them. I know exactly how she felt.

I have a good comeback for people—one you might want to try—when they want me to eat or drink something I don't want or to cheat on my diet. I say, "No, thank you, I like it, but it doesn't like me. It really doesn't agree with my stomach." Then they usually stop.

Sometimes we don't realize how strong the influence of other people can be on our lives.

Sometimes that influence can be brutal, even tragic. The story of my grandmother's neighbor Louise comes to mind.

Louise was beautiful, with a face like that of a porcelain doll. Her voice was soft and soothing, and I will always remember how bright and happy her eyes shined when she laughed. She had a joy of life that was infectious.

Louise loved sharing her life with my grandmother, especially after she got married. From what I was told, Louise's husband was an important businessman. I met him once; he looked like someone had inflated him—large, round, and loud. I really never understood the attraction, but then, I was a kid. What did I know about such things?

At first, Louise looked very happy to have married "the man of my dreams," as she called him, but shortly after her marriage, her demeanor changed. She became anxious and more concerned with her appearance—her hair and her face, but especially her figure. I began to notice that not only were her body and face changing shape, but her eyes no longer had that familiar sparkle. Louise looked as though the life inside of her had drained out.

One day, my grandmother took a basket of fruits and vegetables over to Louise, only to discover later that she had given them to another neighbor. Louise told the neighbor, "I must watch my figure. My husband thinks I am too fat."

I was astonished when I heard that story. Now, I know I was a very skinny kid, but if I stood next to Louise, I looked like the neighbor's cow.

I never saw her again. A few weeks later, I learned the sad news: Louise had committed suicide. I went numb. I could not think or speak; I couldn't even feel the tears streaming down my face. Louise had been so distraught over her husband's constant complaints about her weight and his threats to leave her if she gained even an ounce that she couldn't bear her life anymore. I asked myself, "What depth of inner ugliness would cause a human being to inflict such cruelty upon another person?" Everything she was, beautiful inside and out, he was not.

If you're in a relationship in which the other person is unsupportive or even cruel, trying to sabotage you at every turn or resenting the time you take for yourself, there may be bigger issues brewing under the surface. You may have to examine whether you want to stay in that relationship and whether you want that kind of life. Living with an unsupportive person can make you ambivalent about your health, ambivalent about your goals, and ambivalent about yourself. The changes you need to make may be greater than what you eat or how you exercise. You may need to get out of a destructive relationship, make a break, and move on, or you'll never reach the level you have set for yourself.

I've had to do this once or twice in my own life, so I know what you're faced with. I've been in relationships in which the other person made me feel guilty when I had to practice or play a match when that person wanted to do something else. And my career suffered as a result.

The quality of our relationships matters so much to our well-being. People with a doom-

and-gloom attitude can siphon off your energy, contribute to frustration, and hurt your physical and mental health. If you cling to destructive relationships, it only heaps another burden onto living. Once you get away from the influence of such relationships, you'll find it much easier to make positive lifestyle changes and get your life back in gear again.

When I made my comeback at age 43, I had to deal with a lot of naysayers in the media, in the tennis world, and even in my family. They'd say that I was "tampering with my legacy" and that my glory days were behind me, or they'd suggest that my longevity in the sport was due to a lack of depth in women's tennis. Every single time I did a press conference, I'd always get the questions: "Aren't you too old?" "Do you think you should still be playing?" Often, I still hear people say, "She'll lose because of her age."

People have been putting limitations on me for a long time. First, everybody talked about how I was too young. Then, they talked about how I was too old. For only a very short period of time was I just right in everyone's eyes, including those of the press.

Here's how I see it: You can't let other people set your limitations. You can't go on what anyone else says or does. If I had done that, I would never have left my home country. I would never have broken the records I've broken. I would never have had the chance to play in the Olympics. You would never have heard of me!

People who succeed take chances. They don't listen to negative comments along the way. You have to ignore the naysayers, not let them sabotage you, and go after what is in your heart.

FOLLOWING THROUGH

- Be up-front with people in your life about your commitments. Ask your spouse, partner, family, or friends to help you make healthy lifestyle changes. Tell them you're serious about it, but more important, show them by your actions. Nothing could be truer here than that old saying, "Actions speak louder than words."

- Have a heart-to-heart talk with those who seem to challenge or resist your decision to make changes for a healthier lifestyle. If a friend complains, say something like, "I know I may not seem as much fun, but this is really important to me, and I'd like your support."

- Identify your needs to your friends and family so they are clear as to your direction and your goals, as well as what you need from them to get there. Support is a two-way street, and maybe the people in your life want to live a healthier lifestyle, too. If so, make your support mutual. Team up with a buddy and help each other stay on track. The more help, support, encouragement, and information you share with others, the more positive the results will be for everyone in your life.

- Let the negative people in your life know that their attitude is destructive and that it undermines your relationship with them as well as your health. Go so far as to say that you fear losing the sense of trust you have that they will always be there for you.

- If you're dealing with a spouse or partner

who is negative and unsupportive, suggest that there are ways your fitness program might actually strengthen the bonds between you. You might walk together after dinner, eat healthy meals together, or join a gym together.

- If your partner still doesn't come around, don't give up or give in yet. Seek professional counseling to sort through the issues and re-open the lines of communication. I can't emphasize it enough: Your health as well as your relationship may be at stake.
- Focus on the fun, not the food. Find activities other than eating that you can enjoy with your friends. Instead of meeting for pizza, go to the movies, visit a museum, or take a class together.
- Stand up for yourself. If someone is trying to force food on you, politely—but firmly—decline. Practice saying, "No, thank you; I'm full." Who can argue about whether you've had enough to eat?
- I know that many of you are raising children—kids who probably like to eat sweets, fast food, and other stuff. You have choices, though. You can set an example by eating healthy food and exercising, and hopefully that will convince your family of the benefits of a fit lifestyle. Ask them to join you in making healthy changes; it will be good for them as well. Or you can tell your kids that if they want to eat junk food, they can bring it into the house in single servings or buy it with their own money at the food court.
- Be flexible. Work around any resistance from your family. If they insist on eating fattening food or refuse to skip dessert, try to compro-

mise. Adjust your own portions, explore ways to lighten old favorites, and try a ripe mango (my favorite!) or other fruit as a delicious alternative to a fattening dessert.
- If you don't have an obvious choice for a workout partner, keep looking. It could be a neighbor, co-worker, relative, or the person sitting next to you in that new class you're taking.
- Lighten up. Keep a positive attitude about your commitment, but don't become a food evangelist or try to convert everyone to your program.

Whether your family and friends are supportive or not, it's still up to you to reach your health and fitness goals. They might put up roadblocks, but if you really want to get in the shape of your life, nothing or no one can stop you from doing so.

MAKE A DEAL

People can support you in ways that make it fun for both of you. Here's an example of what I'm talking about. Candy, a tennis official and a friend of mine, has worn many hats over the course of her life.

She has always battled her weight. When she was a child, her right hand was her knife, fork, and spoon, and sweets were her favorite foods—thus her nickname. If any, and I mean any, dish contained anything remotely resembling sugar, she'd eat it. The only reason she ate spaghetti was because the sauce contained sugar. At restaurants, she'd look at the dessert section of the menu first and then move backward.

Ironically, not only was sugar her primary weakness, she also drank huge amounts of sugar-free diet soda. Go figure!

About 6 months ago, a mutual friend, who had been jumping up and down with frustration over Candy's excessive consumption of diet drinks, bet her $1,000 that she could not stay off them for 1 month. This was a fair test, not too long, yet long enough to see if cutting out diet sodas would help what the friend called "memory loss due to shell-shocked neurons."

Candy, who loves challenges, accepted the bet. With the exception of a fat-free chai latte once a week, the only drink permitted was water. (I'm not sure if Candy would have agreed to the bet if it involved sugar and other sweets.)

Swearing off diet drinks wasn't easy at first. In Candy's words, "The first week was like I was on a Freddy Krueger roller-coaster ride. The week started out normal and then got ugly as it progressed. First, I started dreaming I was drinking diet soda, then the soda cans started sprouting hands. Eventually, I was being chased by the diet cans and finally found myself being swallowed up by them."

Candy put her mind to it, and she did it— she had no diet drinks for a whole month. She won the bet, and she thought she could go back to drinking sodas.

As it turned out, the money was the carrot she needed to make some changes. After her month-long break, Candy took a sip of diet cola. She spit it out. "God, what was I thinking!" she said. "This tastes terrible! I wonder how I ever drank so much before; I guess that is why they call some habits an 'acquired taste.'"

It's been 6 months, and water is now her drink of choice. Other things have changed, too. Candy feels more clearheaded. She exercises more. She has even improved her eating habits.

Look at Candy's experience from the vantage point of your own body: Once you clean out your system, little by little, it's as if your body recognizes junk food and processed food as the poisons they are. Once you start getting more active, you'll notice that you feel lethargic if you return to couch potato status. The body revolts, so to speak, and no longer do you want to eat stuff that's not good for you or slump on the couch watching TV day after day. You'll automatically choose habits that make you feel optimally energized and optimally healthy. Once you get into those habits, it's easier to maintain them because of the positive effect they have on your body and the good feelings they bring to your life.

FOLLOWING THROUGH

- Maybe you can make a similar deal with a friend of yours—to lose a certain amount of weight, to stop eating junk food, to do a set amount of exercise each week, to give up alcoholic beverages for a while, or whatever else the stake is. The bet doesn't have to be $1,000; it can be $1. The money doesn't matter; it's the result that matters.
- Have a friendly competition—who can exercise the most times in a given week, who can walk the farthest, whatever you want. The best thing about this type of competition is that everyone is a winner.

FIND COACHES

In the broadest sense of the word, a "coach" is someone who holds you accountable and helps you live up to your potential. I think we all need coaches from time to time because they can make a real difference in our lives as long as they are committed to our success. Anyone who wants to win, and get more out of life, can benefit from having a coach.

Where do you find coaches? For one thing, you don't have to be a world-class athlete to have one. A coach may be someone who has technical expertise or professional training in nutrition, exercise, or any other aspect of health. Nutritionists, personal trainers, exercise instructors, doctors, chiropractors, alternative health care practitioners, therapists in a physical rehab clinic—these are examples of people who could serve as coaches in your life.

Some of the best coaches may be among the people you know best—for instance, a friend or relative with knowledge in a special area to whom you can go for advice, or even your workout partner, from whom you can gain mutual support and information.

A good coach can spot things right away. A nutritionist, for example, can identify where your diet misses the mark. A personal trainer can tell if you're doing an exercise correctly and can help you adjust your form or technique if you're not. If you're not feeling in peak form, a physician can tell you what your symptoms mean and what to do about them. A good coach who is also a friend can do even more for you, like bolster your morale and provide encouragement when you need it. If your moti-

vation flags, you don't have to worry—the coach can inspire you and help you see what you can be rather than what you are.

Every coach has something to offer, and each one can approach a situation a little differently. For example, I've worked with a number of coaches, sometimes two at once. When I worked with Dr. Renee Richards, she was really good at the technical aspects of the game, such as showing me how to jump into my serve for added power and develop my topspin backhand. Mike Estep, on the other hand, was not so much into technique as he was into tactics, mapping out strategy. His advice involved action, whereas Renee's stressed reaction. For example, planning for a match with Chris Evert, Mike would say, "Attack her serve," while Renee's advice was always technical: "Get the ball in play, get the return deep."

Billie Jean King went more into the mental aspect of the game, which people really neglected and didn't go into much back then. We just didn't address it enough.

My current coach, Stefan Ortega, has raised my game a few more notches by working with me on my shots. You see, I don't hit the ball the same way I did 20 years ago or even 3 years ago. When I was a young tennis pro, our serves were timed with one of those radar guns, and mine was clocked at 91 miles per hour—considered pretty fast back then. The women pros today are serving the ball a lot harder and much faster. Among them, Venus Williams has recorded the world's fastest tennis serve, clocked at 127 miles per hour, and I actually hit one at 109.

So how come these girls are hitting the ball

harder than I do, but they're not as strong as I am? In a word, technique. Today's tennis stars, in general, are hitting the ball in new ways not seen in my day. Technique has changed so much; every shot is smacked like a serve, with the utmost power and precision. If I develop the same technique they use, then arguably, I should hit the ball harder and faster because I'm stronger than some of the ones who hit the heck out of the ball. So that's what I'm working on with my coach—changing my technique to get more out of my game. I just love it, too; it's fun to learn new ways to hit the ball.

The main reason we use coaches is to learn from them, and every coach adds something. Very few coaches can look at the whole picture from every angle and cover all the bases. If you talk to different people about the same problem, you'll get slightly different takes on it. It's up to you to figure out which advice works for you and which can really make a difference. My strength has been that I take the advice that I know works for me. I'm open enough to ask people questions and ask for suggestions. People who advise me may tell me 10 things, and I'll use maybe 3 of them.

Keep this in mind: A coach prepares you, but a coach can't do it for you. Achieving your goals, changing your lifestyle—it's ultimately up to you. It's like tennis: If you aren't prepared by the time you're on the court, you may never be.

FOLLOWING THROUGH

- Find "coaches" by getting recommendations from people you trust, even from people in the same field. For example, ask chiropractors who they go to when they need an ad-

justment. Who has a good reputation and who comes highly recommended? Get the answers, and you've found your coaches.

- Join a charity training program such as Team Diabetes (www.diabetes.org) or Team in Training (www.teamintraining.org), which raises money to support the Leukemia and Lymphoma Society. Organizations like these often supply coached workouts in exchange for volunteering to raise contribution pledges.

- Hire a personal trainer for a few sessions to help motivate you and get you going.

- If you need a support system to help you with a weight-loss diet, seek professional expertise from a commercial, hospital-based, or health club–sponsored program.

- Post a sign at work saying you are looking for people to work out with you on your lunch hour, or ask the human resources department about starting a walking club during lunch.

- Ask your workout partner to read up on various subjects relating to health and fitness, and you do the same, so you can count on each other for support.

- Use this book or other resources as a coach. Support is support, no matter where it comes from!

TAP INTO THE HEALING POWER OF SUPPORT

I used to hate being alone. I always needed somebody down the hall or in the same building, or I'd start getting sad and nervous. I don't know why; I just really enjoy having positive people around me—people who make me feel good. I have gotten over my fear of being alone, though it took a long time. Some days, I find that I actually look forward to more free time alone, and I do need shelter when I'm playing tennis. Today, if I'm home alone with a couple of hours to kill, I like it very much. I don't have to schedule anything. I can read, watch television, walk on the beach, dabble in woodworking, or do some remodeling. I admit I'd feel strange, though, if all my dogs weren't there. They don't talk back, and I'm getting to appreciate this more and more.

While it's good to have some alone time—it's a great safety valve when you're under pressure—you don't want to let yourself get too socially isolated. It can be harmful to your health in the long term. Some studies suggest that social isolation is on a par with smoking, high blood pressure, and lack of exercise as a risk factor for getting seriously ill and even dying prematurely.

On a positive note, good friends can add years to your life. A huge body of research shows that when you have strong social contacts—with a spouse, a partner, a close-knit family, a group of good friends, or other people—you're apt to live longer and have better health. Though relationships sometimes go sour and can become counterproductive, having a good support system enhances your immunity, reduces stress, and lifts depression. Good friends—well, let's just say they're good for your health.

FOLLOWING THROUGH

- Volunteer for a charity organization or community cause or work on a political cam-

paign. This can be a great way to meet new people.
- Begin to socialize more with neighbors or co-workers. Invite them over for a social gathering or offer to help them out in a pinch.
- Attend a class to learn something new—and meet new people.

FINALLY . . . LEAD BY EXAMPLE

Once you get your health habits in order, you have the potential within you to bring out the best in others. There are few things more satisfying in life than being a good role model, someone who sets an example and motivates other people toward positive change. A relationship is created, one that has mutual benefits.

For me, this has happened with Stefan, my current coach. At the time he started coaching me, Stefan was at least 20 pounds overweight, he drank a lot of soft drinks, and he smoked a pack of cigarettes a day. Stefan is a great coach, and he made a difference in my game within a few weeks by overhauling my technique. The only drawback was that for him to give me what I needed, which was all of his attention, he had to get healthier because he couldn't keep up. He needed to get in better shape so he could hit the ball with me and have the stamina to stay with me on the court. He knew it, too—that to work hard for me, he had to get in better shape.

I didn't nag him about his habits. I didn't needle him. I just led by example as best I could. Since he's been around me, eating what I eat, he has lost a lot of weight. He drinks water instead of so many soft drinks. He has cut his smoking down to about three cigarettes a day (he has to quit cold turkey if I win a Grand Slam!). His energy level is much higher, and he looks younger. He's 30 years old, but 2 years ago, he looked like he was in his forties.

Best of all, Stefan now feels so much better that he doesn't want to go back to the way he used to be. In the beginning, he felt a need to get in shape. Now it's a want. He *wants* to feel healthy and energetic.

So that's the benefit of a supportive relationship—we contributed something positive to each other in a balanced way, so that we both benefited. I showed him how to eat for health and energy, and in return he was able to give me everything he had, everything I needed. I like the idea that you can give somebody help and get help in return. You work together, and your fitness programs feed off each other. It's all about giving and taking, in a positive way. It's about being a good role model for those around you, and it's about representing yourself in the best possible way.

If you have ever started a diet or fitness program and failed to stick with it, there's a good chance that you didn't have the right mind-set or support firmly in place first. Let me encourage you: If you take the first two steps to heart and mind, you'll have some important ducks in a row.

With the next step, it's time to get your food and nutrition in order. Let's make this the last time you have to struggle with diet-related change!

Chapter 4

Step 3:
Fuel Your Body
and Mind

Food is my friend. It has helped me surpass even my greatest expectations of athletic performance, endurance, and good health.

You look 10 years younger than you did when we first got to the restaurant."

That's what a friend of mine said to me as I was halfway through my meal at a natural foods restaurant in New York City.

Ten years younger? I'm not so sure. But fresh, pure food has remarkable rejuvenating power, inside and outside your body. Not only did I feel better as I ate my meal of spaghetti squash with pesto sauce and a salad and enjoyed my beverage of young coconut juice, but I looked better. All in less than an hour.

Let me back up and tell you the rest of the story. I was in the city for 3 days of work. Exhibitions. A speech. Autograph signings. Cocktail parties. Business and tennis, tennis and business, all crammed into 3 stressful days. I had no time to relax. I was getting very little sleep. I was emotionally spent and physically exhausted. The energy had just seeped out of me, and the signs of strain were etched on my face.

Then, miraculously, one simple meal of fresh, natural food restored me. Think about it: If a single meal could make that much difference, can you imagine how you'd look and feel if you ate that way all the time? Plastic surgery, makeovers, expensive skin creams—who would need them?

The reason I bring up this story is to show you the restorative power of a good diet. The foods I eat have made me feel younger and have given me the stamina to play tennis well past the age when most players have retired. I see no reason why I won't feel the same way 10 years from now.

What I'll tell you about in this step is how I eat, including the foods I enjoy, and how you can begin to adopt some of the same nutritional strategies. In fact, the foods and juices I recommend provide a scientifically sound way to counter the effects of aging and help you maintain a healthy weight and reach new heights of energy and stamina. I didn't always have a handle on how to eat for health and performance, though. My nutritional life has evolved. Now I know what kind of diet I need, and I love what it does for me. I hope it does the same for you.

MY NUTRITIONAL EVOLUTION

For most of my career, I've done things instinctively, like leaving my home country for America, doing whatever seems right, and even knowing what's right to eat for my body. Yes, my nutrition has moved through various stages, including sampling too much junk food when I was a young tennis pro fresh out of the Czech Republic and planted on American soil.

After a while, though, I knew that the days of waiting for intuitive insight into good nutrition were over. I became more sophisticated about sports nutrition in the eighties, when I began a full-time diet and exercise program. I started cutting down on red meat, sugar, fats,

and oils; eating more whole grains, vegetables, fruits, and lean meats and dairy products; having tomato sauce over pasta instead of rich cream sauces; and having chicken grilled rather than fried. I was now eating a lot of whole grain pasta and breads, grains, fish, and chicken and enjoying rice milk on my oatmeal. As someone who loves to eat, I began to experience the joys of this new diet. I could load up on all kinds of goodies, provided they were the right kind. The diet was good for my body, summoning up added power I didn't know I had. This was definitely what you'd call a high-carb diet. I know it helped me to get in the best shape of my career up to that time. From 1982 to 1987, I was able to win six consecutive Wimbledon titles. When you eat better, your "game"—whatever it is for you—will pick up almost right away.

In 1990, I began to think seriously about being a vegetarian because I love animals—which is why I'm surrounded by so many dogs and cats. As an animal lover, I didn't want to eat animals. But every time I tried to be a vegetarian, people kept talking me out of it. Finally, I stopped listening to them and said good-bye to most animal foods, with the exception of eggs and some dairy on occasion. I remained a vegetarian for about 7 years. During that time, I felt good about myself, better than I ever had, because I wasn't eating anything that could walk, run, swim, or fly. I could watch the movie *Babe* and not feel guilty!

Although I liked the "vegetarian me," I eventually had a stamina problem. I struggled to get through a match, practically pooping out midway. I was probably not taking in enough protein

WOMEN, HORMONES, AND DIET

In my early days of playing tennis, I had awful menstrual cramps. I really did not want to do anything but lie doubled over in bed, since back then, there was no ibuprofen to take care of the pain. Also, right before my periods, my coordination could be so off that I didn't even want to drive a car, so you can imagine the effect on my game. I lost more than one match in my career thanks to my period. Of course, most women pros can probably make the same claim.

Once I started controlling my diet, my cramps became minimal, and my coordination wasn't thrown off as much. Also, I stopped being so moody right before my periods, whereas before, I'd always gotten really low in energy and morale. From personal experience, I know that diet and hormones are intricately linked.

At 49, I carry a little more fat around my waist than I did 20 years ago, even though I've been eating pretty much the same way and training all through my career. As women approach their fifties, shifting levels of estrogen alter the distribution of fat and slow down metabolism. Body fat continues to increase, and the fat we carried in our hips, legs, and thighs during our thirties and forties begins to move toward our waistlines.

The question is: Can you compensate nutritionally for this shift? Quite possibly—by adding 1 or 2 servings of soy foods to your diet several times a week. You can get soy in many forms, including soy milk, edamame (steamed soybeans), tofu, and soy nuts. Soy and other vegetables and fruits contain phytoestrogens, plant compounds that appear to mimic estrogen. The

more you eat a plant-based diet, the less trouble you'll have at menopause. This doesn't mean becoming a vegetarian but rather following a diet that emphasizes fruits and vegetables and is low in animal fats.

Also, avoid processed foods at all costs! Eating too many processed foods, such as refined breads, commercial baked goods and sweets, and snacks, upsets the metabolism of insulin in your body, creating a condition called insulin resistance. When you become insulin resistant, your body converts every calorie it can into fat—even if you're trying to lose weight.

Making these dietary changes will go a long way toward balancing your hormones naturally. And don't forget exercise; it's essential for a healthy metabolism.

---

to replace the normal loss of muscle after my matches, and my body was therefore in a chronically worn-down, torn-down state. To make matters worse, I ate some bad eggs, got sick, and could not stomach eggs for years afterward. So I had to liberalize my diet by reintroducing more animal foods into the mix. These supplied the material for muscle repair, and my energy levels shot up fast. It was amazing.

I still eat some fish and poultry, but usually no red meat. People wonder why that is. Besides the philosophical reasons, red meat wipes me out. It feels too heavy in my system. One evening in Aspen—I was in my midthirties then—I had prime rib and a margarita for dinner. The next day, I felt completely deenergized. I know it was the prime rib and not the margarita.

I also avoid red meat because I once had a well-publicized bout of toxoplasmosis caused by eating a hamburger. The illness is caused by a parasite and can be contracted by eating undercooked meat. I realize that these days, meats can be irradiated to reduce harmful bacteria and organisms, but irradiation can degrade the nutritional value of food and may promote the formation of free radicals, nasty molecules in your body that cause disease. So I leave red meat alone—along with other irradiated foods. Irradiating fruit and vegetables to extend their shelf life can mislead you by making old food look fresh. What a sham. I don't want to eat strawberries or any other produce that's a month old! The greater the age of fruit and vegetables, the lower their nutritional value. At least irradiated foods are labeled, so you do have a choice.

If you consider that the centerpieces of my diet have always been fresh fruit and vegetables (preferably organic), my diet hasn't changed much over the past 20 years. My love of fresh foods goes back to my early years. Our family would often go mushroom hunting, then eat some of them fresh and dry and cure the rest in our attic. Also, like every other Czech family, we grew vegetables in our garden at home—but no fruits or nuts. Those we had to buy, although occasionally I would climb a fence in someone's yard and help myself to some cherries or apples. Or I'd snatch apples from the grove that used to be part of my mother's family estate before the Communist takeover of my homeland in 1948. We were never short of nutritious food, so eating healthy is part of my heritage.

MY DIET PHILOSOPHY

These days, people ask me all the time what I eat. Mostly, I try to avoid processed foods. I know they build up the wrong chemicals in my body. The farther a food is from its natural state because of processing (milling, bleaching, frying, and sugaring, or bottling, canning, and other forms of packaging), the more nutrients it has lost. Take whole grains, for example. Most of the grain's nutritive value is found in the outer hull (called the bran) and the germ (such as wheat germ). Yet food manufacturers believe that we prefer bread made from the starchy interior, so they extract the bran and the germ to create milder-flavored but nutritionally inferior white flour. The same goes for rice. It's polished to create a quick-cooking variety with milder flavor, making it devoid of much nutrition.

People have laughed or made faces at my on-the-court eating habits, from the time when I would eat hot dogs or a ham sandwich during the changeovers to today, when I eat energy balls that I buy from an organic market in Miami. The energy balls are made from a mixture of dates, sesame seeds, and walnuts—uncooked and organic. They keep me going at matches, where you sometimes still find players drinking colas, of all things. Tracy, the woman who makes the energy balls, is a former dancer who has a fabulous body and exudes energy. Even from a distance, you can see how healthy she is, and it's mainly because of the kinds of foods she puts into her body.

Sometimes I bring sprout sandwiches onto the court, or various fruit and vegetable juices that I've concocted. The women on the tour look at me like I'm crazy because of the "weird" food I eat. But once I offer a bite to them, they are amazed by how great my food tastes. I swear, if you ate my concoctions before a match and as part of your overall diet, you'd have enough stamina to stay on the court for eight or nine sets against Godzilla.

As for weight-loss diets, I don't go on them. I'm against anything that's too restrictive, including diets that tell you what to eat and what not to eat, so I don't count calories, carbs, or fat. I mainly eat natural, high-quality food and try to avoid a lot of fat and sugar.

I don't eat "artificial" anything. I mean, what's the point? Could a car run on "artificial gas"? I don't think so. If you want to become highly tuned, you need real food that supplies real nutrients.

So what do I define as real food? To show you, let me walk you through a typical day for me.

Upon rising: A piece of fresh fruit or a freshly prepared fruit, vegetable, or fruit-and-vegetable juice.

Breakfast: Eggs sautéed with mushrooms or another vegetable, such as broccoli, or an omelet made with one egg and two egg whites, along with multigrain bread with a little butter or jam; pancakes; or oatmeal—always with a glass of fresh-squeezed juice, such as orange juice.

Lunch: A raw salad, pasta or rice with vegetables, or a vegetable sandwich made with hearty multigrain bread.

Midafternoon snack: A slice of multigrain bread with fresh fruit, such as a banana.

Dinner: Lean protein such as chicken or fish, lots of lightly steamed vegetables, and usually a salad made with a light olive oil dressing.

Evening snack: Fresh vegetable juice.

What I've laid out for you in this book is not a quick-fix "diet." I know that at some point in your life, you've tried some form of diet. Don't be shy; just nod your head a little in agreement. That's great. Now think back to how you felt during that diet. If you're like me, you were, or felt like you were, always thinking about being on a diet. How horrible is that? Not only were you thinking about what you could eat, you were thinking about what you *couldn't* eat. That's a bummer.

In the pages that follow is straightforward information about how to restore and reinforce the natural patterns of eating in your daily life. I've taken what I do and hopefully made it a no-brainer to follow. Once you find out everything these foods can do for you, you'll want to get on board and nourish yourself to superior health. I assure you that even if you make just a few changes to your diet—and do it gradually—you'll look better, feel better, and have the promise of better health.

ORGANIZE YOUR NUTRITION AROUND NATURAL FOODS, INCLUDING RAW FOODS

As you can probably tell, my entire nutritional program is based on eating better-quality foods, including fresh fruits, vegetables, and whole grains. Foods in these categories—which are all plant foods—give you the most nutrients for the fewest calories. In fact, these foods supply most of the vitamins, minerals, fiber, antioxidants, phytochemicals, and enzymes your body needs. If you think you can get away with obtaining these nutrients mostly from supplements and pills, think again! These nutrients are best acquired and assimilated in your body from the whole foods that contain them. Eating a wide variety of these foods will help you achieve top form—and maintain it!

People think that healthy foods like these taste like cardboard. Nothing could be further from the truth. Healthy food can be bursting with flavor; you just have to be imaginative and know how to make it interesting. When you do that, you'll look forward to having it. There's a delicious almond milk smoothie, blended with raspberries and a little maple syrup, that I make for myself. It's heavenly! Every time I drink it, I feel like I'm cheating. Trust me, you can be creative with healthy foods, and to help you, I've included a number of easy-to-fix recipes in Chapter 8.

I also believe it's very important for health and fitness to include some raw foods in your diet. And I'm not talking carrot sticks and celery stalks! I've been to restaurants catering to the raw foods trend that serve a "cake" of raw nuts layered and iced with carob fudge as well as veggie burgers, lasagna, and banana ice cream with chocolate fudge. There's nothing rabbit-like about that menu!

Technically, raw food—sometimes called living food—is a type of vegetarian cuisine using foods that have not been heated above 118°F. Advocates of raw food believe that when foods are heated above that temperature, enzymes in them are destroyed and the foods lose much

of their nutritive value. A basic raw foods diet includes fruits, vegetables, nuts, seeds, and sprouted whole grains eaten in their raw state but prepared very tastily.

No one can deny the wisdom of eating more fruits, vegetables, and other plant-based foods. Enjoying them raw, however, offers some additional health benefits, according to everything I've studied on the subject. For example, eating raw foods:

- Leads to near-automatic weight loss and maintenance, without feelings of hunger or deprivation because raw foods are so filling and naturally delicious.
- Assists in better digestion.
- Can reduce total cholesterol as well as LDL cholesterol (the kind that gums up arteries).
- May reduce the severity of inflammation in conditions such as rheumatoid arthritis.
- Helps normalize blood pressure.
- Allows for higher intake of vitamins A, C, and E, folate, and the minerals potassium and copper than eating cooked foods.
- Helps improve your skin so you start to look younger.
- Leads to increased energy.

Do you have to be a vegetarian or "raw foods faddist" to eat raw food? No way! Eating raw foods all the time would be going to the extreme. Plus, some nutrients are more readily absorbed from cooked foods. For example, you absorb more carotene (a health-building phytochemical) from cooked carrots than from raw carrots, according to studies. As a general rule, just remember that the closer you can get to fresh, whole, natural nutrition, the better your health will be. I know that the more raw food I eat, the better I feel.

According to raw food advocates, the right fruit and vegetable combinations can help you think more clearly and be more mentally alert—especially if those combos are raw, with their nutrients intact. Dark green, leafy vegetables, for example, are rich in calcium and magnesium, two minerals that help nourish your nervous system (of which the brain is a part). The vitamin C in citrus fruits helps your body absorb iron, which has been found to improve concentration and mood. Blueberries contain chemicals that improve brain function, including the ability to remember recent events. Pumpkin seeds are one of the few foods that contain omega-3 fatty acids, which are essential to keep brain cell membranes functioning. Any type of wholesome, unprocessed carbohydrate is great fuel not only for your muscles but also for your brain. Carbs are the chief nutrient fuel for your brain and a great source of thiamin (vitamin B_1), which reinvigorates your brain and nerves.

In Chapter 8, you'll learn how to plan meals that feature health-boosting, brain-building natural foods, including lots of fresh fruits and vegetables. In the meantime, here are some ways to put more fruits and vegetables on your plate.

FOLLOWING THROUGH

- Change the focus of your meals by planning them around vegetables and grains. For example, make plant-based foods at least two-thirds of your meal and lean meat, fish, or low-fat dairy foods less than one-third.
- Populate your diet with plant-based foods that are high in fiber, which keeps your digestive tract in sync and protects against many cancers and other diseases. Beans, lentils, berries, pears, apples, artichokes, avocados, prunes, and figs are among the highest-fiber foods you can eat.
- Experiment with new vegetables and aim for variety.
- Add vegetables to rice or pasta dishes. Some ideas: Add green bell pepper, onion, mushrooms, spinach, or zucchini to spaghetti sauce or add chopped broccoli or spinach to wild rice.
- Stuff a pita pocket with raw or cooked vegetables.
- Add dark green lettuce, mushrooms, and tomato and cucumber slices to sandwiches.
- Keep raw vegetables on hand to eat as snacks or with meals. Serve them alone or with fat-free dips or hummus.
- Instead of meats, top pizza with lots of vegetables, such as tomatoes, onions, green bell peppers, mushrooms, and broccoli.
- Add more vegetables to canned soups or make your own soups with lots of vegetables.
- Add at least one large salad with a light olive oil dressing to your lunch or dinner each day. Use a variety of greens other than iceberg lettuce, which offers very little in the way of nutrition.
- Enjoy fresh fruit for snacks.
- Top pancakes, waffles, or cereal with fresh fruit.

- Have fruit or a fruit salad for dessert.
- Try to have raw fruits and vegetables two or three times a day, with meals or as snacks. Then maybe you can progress to having several raw food meals a week.
- Experiment by trying a few raw food recipes each week. Some of my favorites are included in Chapter 8.

DISCOVER JUICING

If you're aiming for the widely recommended 5 or more servings of fruits and vegetables daily, most experts now advise getting two of them as juices. I've been "juicing" since 1981, and I try to have at least two fresh juices daily, one in the morning and one in the evening.

For me, drinking fresh juices is one of the best ways to get a concentrated amount of quickly absorbed nutrients in order to improve my performance. I've noticed that I'm much more energetic in the morning if I start the day with a fresh juice. One of my favorites is carrot-apple juice made from six large carrots and two apples. One tall glass of that gives my body immediate access to carbohydrates, vitamins, carotenes, minerals, and other performance-boosting nutrients. Juices are also a refreshing way to introduce raw foods into your body.

Here are some of the other important benefits cited by juicing advocates.

- Supplementing your diet with fresh fruit and vegetable juices delivers healing nutrients into your system in a rapid, absorbable manner.
- Because fresh juices are so absorbable, they

promote a healthy digestive system by letting your stomach and intestines rest and regenerate.
- Juicing can be a great weight-loss tool. Fresh juices are nourishing and filling and therefore quell hunger pangs. They are certainly much better beverages than soft drinks, which science says contribute to weight gain and type 2 diabetes.

When I drink a fresh juice, I feel instantly supercharged. You don't really need that cup of coffee to jump-start you in the morning; a fresh juice will do the trick better and give you lasting energy. Besides, caffeine actually blocks the absorption of important minerals such as potassium, magnesium, and phosphorus—nutrients you can get from juice. So put away your coffeemaker and get out your juicer or blender!

Speaking of that, you're probably wondering if you need a lot of fancy appliances to make juice. Juicers, of course, are terrific since they are designed to extract the liquid from a fruit or a vegetable, separating the juice from the pulp. But if you can't invest in a juicer right away, there are alternatives. One is the versatile blender. Unlike a juicer, it liquefies the whole fruit or vegetable into a fiber-filled puree. You can use blenders to make smoothies and make delicious nut milks by blending soaked nuts with water and straining out the nut meal through a sieve. Another alternative is a good citrus juicer, and even the electric models are affordable. With a citrus juicer and a blender, you can make an array of tasty juices and smoothies. (Again, check out my recipes in Chapter 8.)

Once you get in the habit of juicing and see how much better you feel, you may well find that a professional juicer is a vital appliance. It will save you money in the long run, especially considering the prices at most juice bars! I use and recommend the Juiceman line of juicers (www.juiceman.com), particularly the Juiceman Pro. It's made of stainless steel, and its large feeder tube and automatic pulp extraction allow for faster juicing. It can even juice rinds and skins, where the greatest concentration of nutrients can lie. I not only have this juicer on my counter at home, I travel with it wherever I go. One of my first stops whenever I get to a new city is a supermarket or organic food store to stock up on fruits and veggies to juice.

It is much faster than you think to wash and cut up produce and juice it. Not only that, it's fun to experiment with different mixtures of fruits and vegetables. I'm always mixing the ratio and types of fruits and vegetables that I put into my juices. They never taste the same twice, but they're always delicious.

Fresh juices are superior in nutrition and taste to canned, bottled, or frozen juices, but if you don't have time to wash, peel, and chop a bunch of fruits and vegetables, a good option is to have some organically produced juices in your fridge. You can also find a good juice bar in your community where they serve up fresh fruit and vegetable juices and go there regularly.

WHAT SCIENCE SAYS ABOUT JUICES

JUICE	HEALTH BENEFIT
Apple juice	May help prevent declines in thinking that occur as a part of normal aging and in conditions such as Alzheimer's disease
Black currant juice	May help prevent uric acid buildup that leads to kidney stones
Carrot juice	May help boost immunity
Concord grape juice	May promote healthier, wider arteries; helps normalize blood pressure
Cranberry juice	May successfully treat urinary tract infections; may increase blood levels of HDL cholesterol (the good kind)
Juiced ginger (a great addition to any juice)	High in antioxidants; may alleviate mild to moderate nausea; may have anti-inflammatory properties
Orange juice	Supplies antioxidants (nutrients that counter the damaging effects of oxygen in the body) for better immunity against disease
Pineapple juice	Contains a natural enzyme called bromelain that may work as an anti-inflammatory agent
Pomegranate juice	Helps reduce LDL cholesterol in the blood; may promote healthier, wider arteries
Tomato juice	Reduces abnormal blood clotting in people with type 2 diabetes; may help boost immunity

It's best to not limit yourself to one kind of juice, or else you may not get a healthy variety of nutrients. Drink a wide variety of fruit and vegetable juices, smoothies, and nut milks throughout the week. Juices are meant to supplement, not replace, the nutrition you get from whole, fiber-rich fruits and vegetables.

As with anything in life, you can go overboard with juicing. During the 2004 Olympics in Athens, I was drinking a lot of carrot juice in an effort to overcome a sinus infection. I ended up developing carotenemia, a harmless but unsightly condition in which your skin turns orange from absorbing too much of the orange pigment in carrots. You usually can't eat enough carrots to discolor your skin, but if you overdose on carrot juice as I did, you'll start turning orange! Fortunately, the discoloration goes away. At least I learned a good lesson.

One more point along these lines: If you have diabetes, you probably should be careful with fruit juices. A glass of juice is often made from several pieces of fruit, so the carbohydrate content can add up quickly, and the juice may send your blood sugar soaring. Also, anyone who is taking cholesterol-lowering medication should avoid grapefruit juice, which can prevent the drug from being cleared from your bloodstream and allow blood levels to get too high. Check with your physician on these issues.

FOLLOWING THROUGH

- Begin with one glass of fresh juice daily and gradually work up to two glasses.

- Try several simple juice combos (some will require a juicer), such as orange-grapefruit juice (two oranges and one grapefruit), triple citrus juice (two oranges, half a grapefruit, and half a lemon), carrot-apple juice (six carrots and two apples), carrot-beet juice (three carrots and half a beet), apple-pear juice (two apples and one pear), and vegetable tonic (four carrots, two celery stalks, a handful of parsley, and a handful of spinach).
- Use fresh juices to make smoothies. For example, a banana blended with fresh orange juice and a little crushed ice is delicious. There are additional smoothie recipes in Chapter 8.
- If possible, you should drink fresh juices right away to obtain their maximum nutritional benefit, but you can make a batch of juice and refrigerate it for 1 to 3 days before its nutrient quality is lost.
- If you prefer nondairy milks, experiment with making nut milks. They are high in protein and omega-3 fatty acids and are cholesterol-free. Not only that, they're loaded with vitamin E, a powerful antioxidant, and contain minerals such as zinc, magnesium, potassium, calcium, and iron. Nut milks also make a great base for smoothies. I like dairy products, but they don't like me (I get a gassy feeling in my stomach), so I've switched to drinking mostly nut milks.

MAKE WATER COUNT

Millions of us don't feel as good as we should because we don't drink the eight or more glasses of water we need daily. Water is an often overlooked nutrient, one that's involved in practically every bodily process.

I know that if I'm dehydrated, I feel really tired. But when I drink water regularly, I have more energy. That's because water assists in the loading and storage of energy-giving glycogen in the muscles. It's also a solvent and carrier for nutrients. It helps in digestion, circulation, and joint lubrication and even helps decrease the risk of some cancers. It also flushes toxins and metabolic wastes from your system. The more toxins and wastes in your body, the less capable it is of burning fat and losing weight.

There's a guy I've known for a long time who is 6 feet 3 inches tall, big-boned, and age 50-plus. He's also the most overweight person

LIGHTEN UP AT RESTAURANTS

I probably eat out more than most people do because I'm on the road so much throughout the year. It's challenging, I admit, to consistently make healthy choices at restaurants. Here are some tips based on what works for me.

- If you're traveling, scout out healthy restaurants in the city you're traveling to. I do it by researching on the Internet, talking to friends who live in that city, and asking advice from the hotel concierge once I get there.
- Take advantage of the bigger portions in restaurants by saving half of your order for a meal the next day. That's what I do, and it's great!
- Pare down your portions in other ways: Order an appetizer with a side salad, split the meal with a friend, or ask for a half order of the entrée with a double order of veggies on the side as your main course.
- Ask for a doggie bag as soon as the server puts your entrée in front of you. Cut the portion in half immediately and place half of it in the bag, or have the server wrap half of it up for you. If you let it linger on your plate, you may be tempted to finish off the whole thing.
- Get in the habit of asking for salad dressing on the side, or order your salad plain with just a little vinegar or lemon juice.
- Be picky. Ask not only what is in a dish but also how it's prepared. If fats, oils, gravies, or sauces are used, it may not be the smartest choice. Ask for dishes to be prepared in a healthy manner. Restaurants don't have to fry everything!
- Buffets and smorgasbords are challenging! Take only a tablespoon of the various dishes and try not to overload your plate. That way, you won't feel deprived.
- If you feel like having dessert, ask your server for a plate of fresh fruit to top off your meal. Or do what I do: I have two or three bites of a dessert and leave the rest on the table. The waiter sometimes asks, "What's wrong with your dessert?" And I say, "Absolutely nothing. It's delicious." The key is moderation. I enjoy plenty of indulgences, but always in moderation.

WHAT ABOUT NUTRITIONAL SUPPLEMENTS?

You may be surprised to know that unlike many athletes, I don't use supplements or protein powders—with the exception of an electrolyte drink to replace lost electrolytes (minerals) rapidly during a match. I prefer to get my nutrients from food. When eaten intact with their natural food package, nutrients are organized and used much better by your body.

In professional tennis, as in other sports, athletes are drug tested. Nutritional supplements may affect the outcome of those tests through contamination of the product itself, or the nutrient may be metabolized within the body to show up as a drug. You can't take any supplements because there's always a chance they will trigger a positive result on a drug test.

Certainly, there are people who are deficient in calcium or magnesium or who need more vitamin E, vitamin A, or whatever. It's tricky. Some nutrients are really difficult to get through diet alone. But if you're deficient in something and you look at your diet and improve it, you'll balance yourself out in a month with better food. I think it's reasonable for the general population to take supplements as a backup to good nutrition, but it's not wise for drug-tested athletes.

In sport, you have to present as clean an image as possible so people can say you achieved your status through hard work, not because you're taking some chemical agent that makes you stronger. Taking performance-enhancing substances is not wise; it's not good for athletes, and it's not good for the sport. Not only that, but athletes who go down that path are cheating.

I've ever met. He once weighed around 210, but now he tips the scale at 500 pounds. He also has hyperinsulinemia—meaning he has high levels of insulin in his blood—which makes him prone to heart disease and diabetes and keeps him heavy, since insulin is a fat-storage hormone. His diet basically consists of meat and potatoes and diet soda by the gallon, and he gets no exercise. But in all the years I've known him, he has refused to drink water. Once I asked him why. It turns out that he hates the taste of plain water, and he says he'd have to be "desperate" to drink it.

Since metabolism is a chemical process requiring adequate water, and he doesn't drink it, every system in his body has become sluggish. He has no energy. His thinking is muddled. His body can't burn fat effectively. While it's true that many factors figure into these problems, his refusal to drink water is certainly a bad influence on his metabolism.

Keeping your body well hydrated is important for preventing dizziness, cramps, and exhaustion during exercise, too. It's generally a good idea to drink 1 to 2 cups of water 2 hours before you exercise, then drink more during your workout. When I work out, I drink a few ounces of water for every 10 minutes that I exercise. After your workout, you should replace the water you've lost through perspiration—

about 2 cups of water for each pound of lost body weight. If you can make the commitment to start drinking more water, you'll definitely notice a change in the way you feel and in your energy, and you'll feel the mental kick that sufficient water gives.

Try this with me: In the morning, instead of your usual cup of coffee or tea or can of cola, drink a glass of cold water. Supposedly, drinking cold water gives a little boost to your metabolism since your body burns calories to warm up the water. Then take a minute to notice how rejuvenated you feel.

I prefer to drink bottled water, mainly because it's easy to take with me, and I really don't like the taste of tap water. Bottled water fits my needs and my lifestyle. I am very picky when it comes to water; let's just say I'm spoiled.

There are different types of bottled water, so it helps to read labels. Spring water, for instance, comes from an underground formation from which water naturally flows to the Earth's surface. Purified water has been processed to remove minerals and contaminants; distilled water is one example. Some purified water is actually purified tap water, and the label must state that it comes from a municipal water supply.

Mineral water contains naturally occurring minerals and trace elements. In other words, these are in the water at its source and can't be added later. Sparkling bottled water, which I often enjoy with a meal, has a bit of a fizz caused by the carbon dioxide it contains. Artesian water is taken from an aboveground well that taps an aquifer, a water-bearing layer

of rock or sand. Well water comes from a hole bored, drilled, or otherwise constructed in the ground to tap the water aquifer. All bottled water is strictly regulated at the federal level by the FDA and at the state level by state agencies.

Tap water can be contaminated with lead found in household plumbing materials, nitrate from fertilizers, disease-causing microbes that pass undetected through filtering systems, and other pollutants. In fact, I've read that there are 85 possible contaminants that can get into drinking water, according to the EPA. Fortunately, though, because of the federal Safe Drinking Water Act, municipal water systems serving 25 people or more are constantly tested for harmful substances. If there is a problem with your water supply, you'll be warned through the media or other outlets.

On the whole, Americans have good, clean drinking water. You can get information about your community's water supply by logging on to www.epa.gov and following the proper links. Filtering out contaminants from tap water with a home water filter is another good option for making sure your drinking water is safe.

FOLLOWING THROUGH

- Drink a glass of water upon rising in the morning, one to two more before lunch, and more before dinner and during exercise. We need at least eight 1-cup servings, or 64 ounces, of water a day.
- Sip water in your car on the way home from work.

- The next time you pick up lunch at the local deli, reach for bottled water rather than a soda.
- Buy or use 16- or 24-ounce bottles rather than 8-ounce ones. Then you can track how many bottles you need each day.
- If you don't like the taste of plain water, try adding some fresh lemon or lime, cucumber slices, or fresh mint for a refreshing new taste.
- Be sure to drink plenty of water when traveling by air, since airplane cabins are notoriously dry, and you can become dehydrated.

THERE'S ALWAYS ROOM FOR A LITTLE MORE ADVICE

It's easy to give advice, and I've just given a whole chapter's worth on nutrition. I believe we were designed for a diet of freshness, a back-to-nature way of eating that gives us a shot at what we all want: maximum health. It shouldn't be surprising, then, that when we stray from that path and eat poor-quality food, the detour, in large part, is the root of illness and poor health. The first time I recognized this truth in big, bold, living color was when a longtime friend, Joyce, told me the story of twins, Carla and Carmella, whom she met while traveling to and from work in New York City.

Joyce first became acquainted with the twins during a subway ride uptown, and they often sat together, squashed like sardines in the very compact tin can of a train. Many times, the train would come to a halt, and they'd have to wait for it to move again. On one occasion, the train was stuck in a tunnel for more than 40 minutes. There wasn't much to do but look through the windows into the dark tunnel or talk with those around you, so that's what she and the twins did—talk, about anything and everything.

What confused Joyce about the twins was that they looked like anything but. Carmella looked like Carla's much-older sister rather than her twin, even though both were 30 years old. Eventually, Joyce learned why.

One afternoon on the subway, Carla explained that as an infant, she became seriously allergic to mainstream infant nourishment. When she was old enough to eat whole foods, her pediatrician made sure she followed a diet of fresh fruits, vegetables, and limited types of protein. She became accustomed to that way of eating and made it a habit for the rest of her life. Carmella, on the other hand, could eat "anything," and usually did.

As the two grew up, Carmella became a fast-food junkie, which resulted in weight gains that sometimes tipped the scale toward obesity. Carmella tried every diet imaginable but could never stay on any of them longer than a few days here or there. The ups and downs of her weight, coupled with her poor eating habits, eventually took a severe toll on her health. She developed kidney disease. Ignoring the warnings of her doctor, Carmella continued to eat fast food, junk food, and all sorts of processed foods.

A year later, one of her kidneys failed and had to be removed. Her doctor, sister, and friends pleaded with her to change her dietary habits, but to no avail.

Within 3 years of the first kidney problem,

WILL EATING THIS WAY HELP ME LOSE WEIGHT?

Losing weight is really a matter of simple math. You have to eat fewer calories than you burn through normal activity and exercise. If you follow the guidelines here, you'll hardly have to count calories.

The foods I emphasize are nutritionally dense, meaning they supply loads of nutrition with relatively few calories while helping you feel full and satisfied. Eating more fruits, vegetables, and high-fiber whole grains will trigger weight loss. But you must be mindful of your portion sizes (especially at restaurants where everything is supersized). Each portion of lean meat, poultry, or fish, for example, should be about the size of the palm of your hand, and each vegetable, fruit, or grain portion should be the size of your fist. Use good fats such as olive oil or flaxseed oil—but no more than 1 or 2 tablespoons a day.

Carmella's other kidney began to fail. She started dialysis twice a week, increasing to three times a week less than 2 months later. She was on the donor list for a new kidney, but no donor was forthcoming.

As you might imagine, Carmella's health and spirits began to decline. Carla stepped in and made a "twin decision." She would give up one of her kidneys, but only for a price: Carmella had to change her entire way of eating for the rest of her life. Carla didn't want to be "twinless," but she also wasn't going to give up her kidney if Carmella wouldn't promise to take care of it.

Carmella accepted; she showed a kind of determination Carla had never seen before, and she began a physician-monitored diet in preparation for surgery. Immediately after receiving her sister's kidney, she willingly followed a very closely monitored series of health changes, including diet, exercise, and what she called "a real attitude adjustment."

There is a happy ending: Now in their early fifties, both are doing well. Instead of looking like different-aged sisters, they now look more like the twins they are—identical, almost.

I bring up this story not as a scare tactic, because those don't work anyway. I just want to remind you that you are a person of value, and one of the best ways to support that self-worth is by honoring yourself through healthy choices and habits.

I realize that none of us, including me, is perfect, with the willpower to stick to something 100 percent day in and day out. I cheat on my program a little anyway, because I try to not overdo anything. Even so, when I made the effort to eat more fruits and vegetables, my health and my vitality—which were good to begin with—just got that much better. The foods you eat should be a power source, not an energy drain, so try making these changes, even if it's just for a week. You won't regret it.

When I finally got my diet straightened out, I became interested not only in nutrition but also in "food quality"—where the food was grown, how it was harvested, and whether it was treated with pesticides or antibiotics. I came to be aware that there was a lot of stuff going into food, even fruits and vegetables, that was not a natural part of the food—stuff that isn't good for you and in fact could make you sick. That's when I got interested in organic food, back when it was nothing more than a fad. Today, though, organics aren't just a fad. They're here to stay, and I'm glad. In the next step, you will learn how going organic can take your nutrition and health up a few more notches.

CHAPTER 5

STEP 4:
GO ORGANIC

I don't want to eat anything I can't pronounce.

All the time I was growing up, I would pick apples, cherries, and other fruits right from the trees. I would eat as many as I wanted and give the rest to my friends. I didn't have to wash or peel the fruit because it was so fresh, clean, wholesome, and naturally full of flavor.

After I came to America, I noticed that a lot of the fruits and vegetables in grocery stores were so coated with waxy material and other gunk that water beaded on them. I had to start peeling everything. It was hard to find a tomato that really tasted like a tomato or a cantaloupe that melted in your mouth the way it should. That's when I decided to pay more attention to where I was buying my produce, so I looked for better sources and discovered organically grown foods, sold in health food stores and farmers' markets. I went organic long before the organic foods movement got formalized around 1985. For as long as I can remember, I've gone to health food stores because I like the atmosphere there. They are very peaceful and clean, and the people who work there generally have a great energy about them.

Organic food, by definition, is food produced without pesticides, synthetic (or sewage-based) fertilizers, or hormones and antibiotics. Pesticides in particular are designed to kill, so why would anyone want to put that kind of stuff in their body?

Since becoming more informed about organic foods, I've learned that they are generally healthier than conventionally grown foods. Studies show that organic food is simply more nutritious than conventionally grown food. For example, it's higher in:

- Vitamin C.
- Minerals. On average, organic produce contains significantly higher levels of 21 different minerals.
- Antioxidants and phytochemicals (natural substances in plants that protect against disease).
- Omega-3 fatty acids. Organic milk, for example, has been shown to be 71 percent higher in these beneficial fats than non-organic milk. This research is important, particularly if you consider that many people don't eat enough oily fish to get the benefits of omega-3 fats, which are known to help fight heart disease, diabetes, depression, and arthritis, among other diseases.

Part of the reason that conventionally grown foods have fewer nutrients has to do with the soil in which this food is grown. Soil has been depleted of nutrients due to intensive modern agricultural practices, and what grows in it suffers as a result.

Many people prefer organic foods because they say they taste better. I'm one of them. From personal experience, I've found that fruits and vegetables, in particular, taste better in certain regions of Europe, Australia, and Asia, where organic farming has widely transformed agriculture, making a positive impact on both human health and the environment. Organic farming uses good soil management techniques, natural pest control, natural materials to maintain soil nutrients, and other measures to preserve soil fertility and ecological health. Good soil quality contributes to high food quality—which is why I've become a crusader for all things organic.

There are many ways you can improve the shape of your life, particularly in nutrition, and choosing organically grown foods is one of the most important. You can't really argue with the evidence. You'll definitely be on to something when you begin "going organic." Here's a look at how you can get started.

ORGANIZE YOUR DIET AROUND ORGANIC FOODS

Once you make the decision to retool your diet with more fresh fruits, vegetables, whole grains, and lean meats, seek out and purchase organic foods. One of the main rationales for doing this is to ensure that you eat foods that are not treated with pesticides, additives, and other chemicals.

My opinions are fairly well formed on many things, and food quality (or lack of it) is one of them. I have always been interested in issues relating to food and the environment and have read extensively on these subjects for many years. I'm not afraid to speak my mind on all this, either. I was appalled when I found out that not only can pesticides be found on the surface of produce, but they also seep inside the fruit or vegetable and thus can't be removed by peeling or washing. Some apples are sprayed 16 times with 36 different pesticides! Some of these pesticides are formulated so that their residues are resistant to being washed off by rain or water. This is pretty unpleasant to think about, but important to bring up: The EPA ranks pesticide residues among the top three environmental cancer risks.

I guess I'm waving a flag and taking a stand here: Eating organic is your best defense against polluted, less pure food. Almost all pesticides and residues of pesticides are prohibited in organic foods, and only about 30 "additives" are permitted for use in them. Generally, an additive is a substance put into a food to improve its nutrition, preserve its quality, or flavor or color the food. Any additive or ingredient already linked to allergic reactions, headaches, asthma, growth retardation, hyperactivity in children, heart disease, and osteoporosis is prohibited in organic foods, according to organic standards. In contrast, more than 500 additives are allowed in nonorganically processed foods.

As for meat and dairy foods, unless the products you buy are labeled "organic," you can be fairly sure the animal your food came from was fed an abundance of antibiotics as well as artificial growth hormones and other drugs. While vacationing in South Dakota one year, I had to take one of my dogs into the veterinarian to have her nails clipped. This particular vet treated mostly cattle and other livestock. Seated in the waiting room, I was shocked by all the products lining the shelves: pills for udder infections, ear infections, and hoof and mouth problems. Even more eye-opening were the injectable antibiotics and hormones. I mean, the syringes were as big as rolling pins, with needles just as long. I didn't understand it. I kept thinking to myself, "This cannot be safe for the food supply!"

With organically reared livestock, the use of drugs to fatten up animals and make them grow is not allowed. Some scientists believe that the practice of giving antibiotics to animals encourages the growth of drug-resistant bacteria. That means ever-increasing doses of antibiotics may be required to cure a disease, and some drugs may not work at all. The excessive use of

POTENTIAL ADVERSE EFFECTS OF PESTICIDES

Anxiety	Immune system suppression	Nausea
Convulsions	Indigestion	Poor memory
Depression	Lack of energy	Skin problems
Diarrhea	Loss of coordination	Tremors
Headache	Muscle weakness	Vomiting

Source: Soil Association, Organic Farming, Food Quality and Human Health: A Review of the Evidence, 2001.

antibiotics on factory farms is believed to be connected to a rise in antibiotic resistance in humans, too.

If you eat meat, I suggest that you shop for meat from organically reared animals. What this means is that the animals have been raised and processed in a healthy, humane way. Animals that are "free range," for example, are allowed to roam and graze on local vegetation. This is in contrast to factory-farmed livestock, which are penned in crowded cages with no space in which to move and whose feedlots are sprayed heavily with pesticides to control flies. What's more, these animals are eating produce grown with pesticides. All of this means that pesticides can end up in the meat you eat.

Another important point is that organically reared animals feed on a natural grassy diet. They're not given feed made up of parts of other animals—a practice that has been implicated in mad cow disease.

So please protect your health with organic foods! As I mentioned earlier, they don't have to be expensive, especially when you buy them from places such as Whole Foods, Trader Vic's, Trader Joe's, Wild Oats, and local farmers' markets. These markets sell fresh produce, organic meats, and other foods. Other ways to save bucks on organic food include buying beans, grains, lentils, and nuts in bulk; purchasing organic fruits and vegetables at the peak of their growing seasons (when they're the cheapest); and freezing organic produce so you can

COMPARATIVE PESTICIDE LEVELS IN FRUITS AND VEGETABLES

HIGHEST LEVELS OF RESIDUES	LOWEST LEVELS OF RESIDUES
Apples	Avocados
Apricots	Bananas
Bell peppers, green and red	Broccoli
Cantaloupe	Brussels sprouts
Celery	Cauliflower
Cherries	Corn
Cucumbers	Grapes (U.S., Mexico)
Grapes (Chile)	Green onions
Green beans	Onions
Peaches	Plums
Pears	Sweet potatoes
Potatoes (U.S.)	Watermelon
Spinach	
Strawberries	
Winter squash (U.S.)	

Source: Organic Consumers Organization.

GOING ORGANIC AT RESTAURANTS

I hope that as you begin to buy organic food and experience its superior taste and quality, you'll want to question where more of your food comes from, even when eating at restaurants. One of the most positive trends happening right now is the increase in organic restaurants all over the world as well as in organic items on menus.

Here are some suggestions to help you go organic when you eat at restaurants.

- Locate vegetarian and raw foods restaurants. These establishments generally serve organic foods, but be sure to ask. Organic doesn't necessarily mean "vegetarian," however, and vice versa. It just means that each food used in a dish has the added advantage of being organic, so the meals are free of pesticides, antibiotics, hormones, and genetic modifications.
- Find directories on the Internet that can help you locate organic restaurants. A good place to start is www.localharvest.org, where you can find all of the farmers' markets, family farms, local produce markets, stores that sell grass-fed meats, and other sources of organically grown food in your area.
- Look for "certified organic restaurants." This is a special designation given by an official organic association of a country, proving to consumers that the foods served are truly organic.

---

buy it at a reasonable price and have it year-round.

FOLLOWING THROUGH

- Purchase foods that are labeled "Certified Organic." This means the item has been grown according to strict uniform standards that are verified by independent state or private organizations. Certification tests include inspections of farm fields and processing facilities, detailed record-keeping, and periodic testing of soil and water to ensure that growers and handlers are meeting the standards that have been set.
- Buy organic in-season foods from your local market for the best assurance of pesticide-free produce. You'll find an extensive list of organic foods and products in "Good Sources of Organic Foods" on page 66.
- Look into using commercial vegetable and fruit washes, which are formulated to remove chemical residue from produce. Examples are Environné and Vitanet, available at health food stores and some supermarkets. Or make your own wash by mixing a solution of half vinegar and half water. Swirl foods such as grapes, strawberries, green beans, and leafy vegetables in the wash for 5 to 10 seconds, then rinse with lukewarm water. For other fruits and vegetables, use a soft brush to scrub the food with the solution for 5 to 10 seconds, then rinse with lukewarm water.
- Peel fruits and vegetables known to have high residue levels (see "Comparative Pesticide Levels in Fruits and Vegetables"), but be aware that residues can permeate the food.

(continued on page 68)

GOOD SOURCES OF ORGANIC FOODS

FOOD	MANUFACTURERS/PRODUCTS
Beans	All Eden beans and legumes, including Organic Black Soy and Organic Seasoned; beans (garbanzo/chickpeas, red kidney, pinto, black turtle, adzuki, mung, great Northern, cannellini, lima); lentils (red, green, brown); peas (split, split yellow, black-eyed/cow)
Breads	Big Kitchen, French Meadow Bakery, Garden of Eatin' (blue corn and corn tortillas), Lundberg Rice Cakes, Manna, New Pioneer Co-Op (farm, olive farm, raisin pecan, sourdough, wheat)
Cereals and grains	Arrowhead Mills, Barbara's Bakery, Bob's Red Mill, Country Choice Naturals, Dr. McDougall's Right Foods, all Eden grain products, Erewhon, Golden Temple, Kashi Go Lean!, Lundberg Family Farms, Nature's Path, New Organics, The Organic Garden
Dairy products*	Harmony Hills Dairy, Horizon Dairy, Morningland Dairy, Organic Valley Dairy, Radiance Dairy, Straus Family Creamery
Flours	Arrowhead Mills white rice, kamut; all Eden flours, including organic golden amber durum wheat, amaranth, barley, buckwheat, farina, garbanzo/chickpea, millet, oat, rice, rye, spelt, wheat, oat bran, wheat bran
Frozen foods	Cascadian Farms organic broccoli, corn, plain vegetables, raspberries, blueberries, strawberries; Sno-Pac organic vegetables
Juices	Organic with no vitamins added (check labels carefully): After the Fall Vermont Harvest Moon apple cider, grape juice; Crofters guava, strawberry, papaya, raspberry, apricot, pink lemonade; Eden organic apple, tomato, cherry; Kedem 100% pure grape; Knudsen cherry, grape, mango, pear, strawberry; Mountain Sun organic strawberry, peach, blueberry, cranberry; Santa Cruz ginger, apricot, cherry, raspberry, apple
Nut and fruit butters	Arrowhead Mills certified organic peanut butter, sesame tahini; Eastwind peanut, cashew, tahini, almond; Eden organic apple butter; Joyva sesame tahini; Maranata roasted pistachio, roasted filbert, roasted sunflower, roasted almond; Maranata sesame tahini, cashew, almond; Once Again hazelnut; Sahadi sesame butter; Santa Cruz organic apple-apricot sauce, applesauce; Westbrae Natural Foods raw sesame tahini, toasted tahini
Nuts and seeds	Almonds, Brazil nuts, cashews, hazelnuts, macadamias, peanuts, pecans, pine nuts, pistachio nuts, pumpkin seeds, sesame seeds, sunflower seeds, walnuts
Olive oils (extra virgin)	Alessi Olio, Da Vinci (and extra light, 100% pure), Eden selected, Filippo Berio (and extra light), Gourmet Aritrian, Grey Poupon, L'estornell, Odd Monk, Olitalia, Peloponnese, Spectrum Organic Products, Tassos

FOOD	MANUFACTURERS/PRODUCTS
Other oils	Eden organic sesame, toasted sesame, hot pepper toasted sesame, safflower; Loriva sesame oil; Olitalia grapeseed oil; Sigg grapeseed oil; Spectrum Organic Products natural almond, apricot kernel, avocado, safflower, walnut
Pasta/noodles	Eden, Millina's Finest, Vita Spelt
Pasta sauces	Eden spaghetti sauce, pizza-pasta sauce; Garden Valley organic; Millina's Finest organic; Muir Glen organic
Salad dressings and condiments	Annie's Farmhouse maple mustard, Cascadian Farm organic sauerkraut, Cross and Blackwell capers, Earth Fire Products chutney, Eden organic mustard and imported condiments, Eden organic sauerkraut, Jaffa Gold lemon juice, Krinos imported grape leaves, Melinda extra-hot sauce, Muir Glen organic tomato ketchup, Sandhill mustard, Santa Barbara Olive Company California ripe large or jumbo pitted olives, Spectrum Organic Products zesty Italian dressing
Salsas	Garden Valley Naturals, Muir Glen, New Bounty Organic, Parrot
Sweeteners	Eden organic malted grain sweeteners, Kogee organic cane sugar, organic cane sugar (available from Wholesome Foods and Florida Crystals), Pure USA Honey, Sucanat North America
Syrups	Anderson's pure maple syrup, Cary's premium maple syrup, Eden organic malted grain sweeteners, Hauke Honey pure maple syrup, Spring Tree pure maple syrup, Wholesome Foods organic blackstrap molasses
Teas	Alvita; Celestial Seasonings (except vitamin-enriched teas); Choice organic; Eden Great Eastern Sun; Long Life organic; Maharishi Ayurveda Vata, Pitta, and Kapha churnas and teas and Raja's Cup; Traditional Medicinals; Yogi Organic
Tofu/tempeh/soy/miso	American Pride tofu; Earth Fire Products; Eden products; White Wave organic wild rice tempeh, five-grain tempeh, soy tempeh, sea veggie tempeh, organic tofu
Vinegars	Da Vinci balsamic; Eden apple cider; L'estornell River Run hot pepper; Spectrum Organic Products raspberry wine, red wine, white wine
Miscellaneous	Duchy Originals, Eden soy milk, Imagine Organic Original Rice Dream, Kogee organic nondairy creamer, Mrs. Denson's cookies, Walker's shortbread

*The dairies listed state that all of their products are made with 100 percent organic ingredients. Their animals are not treated with hormones and are fed only organically grown feed. There are no bioengineered dairy cultures or enzymes in their products.

Source: Mothers for Natural Law; www.safe-food.org.

- Consider growing some of your own produce. Bell peppers, tomatoes, spinach, and cucumbers are pretty easy to grow, even in a small backyard garden. Sprouts can be grown indoors, as can herbs. They will flourish on your windowsill and burst with flavor and freshness.
- To reduce your risk of exposure to drugs and hormones used in meat and other animal foods, eat meats in moderation and make sure they're well cooked. Eat the leanest muscle meat possible rather than fatty meats or liver. (Hormones and toxins tend to congregate in the liver and fat of animals.)

BE AWARE OF GENETICALLY ENGINEERED (GE) FOODS

Something else that has really shocked me is the trend toward genetically engineering foods, a process in which the genetic blueprint of a living plant or animal is altered by changing its DNA. This is done by removing the genes from one organism, say a plant, an animal, or a microbe, and inserting them into another in order to produce potentially useful new characteristics, such as resistance to pests or greater crop yields.

Giant chemical companies are the ones doing this work. Here's an example: By splicing three foreign genes—two from the daffodil and one from a bacterium—into rice plants, one company is creating a new form of rice that is high in beta-carotene, which the body converts into vitamin A. This "golden rice" is being given to people in developing countries, where many go blind because their diets don't supply enough vitamin A. But according to the environmental watchdog group Greenpeace, an adult would have to eat at least 12 times the average of 300 grams of rice daily to get the daily recommended amount of vitamin A. Put another way, you'd have to eat about 8 pounds of cooked rice a day in order to get enough vitamin A if golden rice were your only source of the nutrient.

Genetically altered rice isn't the answer, since one food can't—and shouldn't—repair all the damage caused by malnutrition. There's a profit motive behind this, even though the company claims their aim is preventing blindness: They can patent the genetically engineered genes of a seed, then sell the seeds and gain control of the market share in the countries where they sell them. I hate it that food has become so much about profit and politics and less about promoting good health.

What genetic engineering involves is pretty frightening, based on what I've read on the subject. This is just sick—and sickening. Take a look.

- Pigs with human genes
- Tomatoes with fish genes
- Potatoes with jellyfish genes (so the plants glow in the dark when they need to be watered!)
- Vegetables with scorpion genes

Are genetically engineered foods even safe to eat? Scientists who oppose GE foods say that the new genes may produce toxins in the modified food, that the new genes may make a protein that triggers an allergic reaction in some-one who eats the food, or that cancer-causing molecules may be synthesized.

If you live in the United States, more than half the groceries in your shopping cart could contain the products of genetic engineering, but you'd never be aware of it because they aren't labeled. Again, I don't know about you, but I want to know, and I think we have the right to be informed about whether a food is genetically engineered. I'd like to have a choice—please! Mark it "genetically altered," and people will see what they are buying. I will stand up to insist on laws to label these foods.

In the meantime, here are some steps you can take to avoid any unknown consequences of genetically engineered foods.

FOLLOWING THROUGH

- Eat a diet of mostly organically grown foods. By organic standards, inserting genes into living foods is prohibited. Genetically engineered foods can't be labeled as organic.
- Educate yourself on which food companies produce and distribute organic foods. The information in this chapter will help get you started.

KNOW WHAT YOU'RE EATING

If you could see what goes into some foods, you'd never eat them. There are more than 3,000 chemicals put into our foods. I pay very close attention to what I put in my body, so I read labels carefully. I'm really cautious about eating foods with too many preservatives in them, for example. Some medical experts believe that preservatives, in addition to food-coloring agents and flavor enhancers, create an environment in which the immune system begins to react against the additives and consequently triggers allergic reactions. I just don't want to take any unnecessary chances and risk possible side effects. Who knows what half of these hard-to-pronounce chemicals are, anyway? My English is pretty good, but I don't want to eat anything I can't pronounce!

I've read that there are so many preservatives in our modern diet that undertakers report that human bodies do not decompose after death as quickly as they used to. While I can't guarantee the accuracy of that story, I can tell you that it gives me cause for concern.

FOLLOWING THROUGH

- Get in the habit of reading the lists of ingredients on food labels. A good rule of thumb: Choose foods with shorter ingredient lists; the longer the list, the more likely it is that the product is full of additives, preservatives, and artificial colors.
- Watch out for the word *wheat* in product names when buying bread or pasta. Unless the ingredient list includes whole wheat flour as one of the first ingredients, chances are the product is really low in fiber and nutrition.
- Pay attention to whether the flour you buy, and the flour in the bread you buy, is bleached or unbleached. Bleached flours not

ADDITIVES TO AVOID

ADDITIVE	USE IN FOOD	POTENTIAL RISKS
Acesulfame potassium	Artificial sweetener permitted only in foods such as sugar-free baked goods, chewing gum, gelatin desserts, and soft drinks	Poorly tested; two animal studies suggest it may cause cancer
Blue 1	Artificial coloring used in beverages, candy, and baked goods	Poorly tested; suggestions of small cancer risk
Blue 2	Artificial coloring used in pet foods, beverages, and candy	Suggestions of brain tumor risk in an animal study
Olestra	Indigestible synthetic fat	Can cause diarrhea and loose stools, abdominal cramps, flatulence, and other adverse effects; reduces body's ability to absorb certain cancer-fighting nutrients
Potassium bromate	Used to increase volume of bread and produce bread with fine crumb	May cause cancer in animals; banned virtually worldwide except in Japan and the United States
Propyl gallate	Preservative used in vegetable oil, meat products, potato sticks, chicken soup base, chewing gum	Animal studies suggest cancer risk
Red 3	Artificial coloring used in cherries in fruit cocktail, candy, and baked goods	Evidence suggests it causes thyroid cancer in rats; FDA review committee in 1983 recommended a ban but was overruled
Saccharin	Artificial sweetener used in dietetic foods or as tabletop sugar substitute	Linked in animal studies to cancer of the bladder, uterus, ovaries, skin, blood vessels, and other organs
Sodium nitrite/ nitrate	Preservative, coloring, flavoring used in bacon, ham, frankfurters, lunchmeats, smoked fish, and corned beef	Studies link various types of cancer to consumption of cured meat and nitrite by children and pregnant women and other adults
Yellow 6	Artificial coloring used in beverages, sausage, baked goods, candy, and gelatin	Animal tests suggest that this dye (the third most widely used) causes adrenal gland and kidney tumors; may also cause occasional allergic reactions

Source: Center for Science in the Public Interest; www.cspinet.org.

only have had the bran and germ removed, they are also lower in protein, vitamins, and minerals. Some bleached flours have also been whitened with chemicals and contain potassium bromate, banned in some countries and known to cause cancer in animals.

■ Be familiar with common adverse additives. With so many chemicals being used in food production, it's virtually impossible to keep track of every possible risk. The chart "Additives to Avoid" is based on information from the Center for Science in the Public Interest, a watchdog group that monitors food quality and safety. The chart lists additives we should definitely avoid because they have either been inadequately tested or may be unsafe in the amounts normally consumed. The bottom line: The next time you pick up something to eat, ask yourself if you really know what's in it.

GO ORGANIC IN OTHER WAYS

I've long been passionate about cleaning up the environment that we have so successfully polluted. In 2004, when exposure to mold (on my luggage, of all places!) made me really sick with a sinus infection, headache, and sore throat, I was alerted to the fact that our personal environment—home or office—can be just as polluted as the outside environment. I've gotten aggressive about making sure my surroundings support my health, and I take things like indoor pollutants seriously because I know they can lead to health problems, especially in susceptible people.

Our bodies, thankfully, are designed to filter out and eliminate many toxins. Yet if we're overexposed to chemicals in the environment, our bodies may respond with illness in the form of breathing problems, headaches, allergies, and, in extreme cases, cancer. These days, the use of household and garden chemicals and personal care products is at an all-time high. Although the individual ingredients in them are approved as safe for use, we just don't know what long-term exposure to all of them may do to our health. Once they are poured down the drain or onto our lawns, they may make their way into the water supply or otherwise harm the environment. Fortunately, there are some simple measures you can take to guard your health and protect the planet at the same time.

FOLLOWING THROUGH

- Look for personal care products labeled "organic," which are likely to be made with botanicals, vitamins, and other natural ingredients. Since most of these products end up going down the drain and into the water supply, I prefer those with fewer synthetic substances. How can I tell? If the ingredient list on the back of the product includes a lot of hard-to-pronounce chemical names, I keep shopping around.

- Reduce your exposure to fluoride. This is one of the most toxic chemicals in our environment, more toxic than lead and only slightly less toxic than arsenic, according to a handbook called *Clinical Toxicology of Commercial Products*. Fluoride can build up in your body over time, possibly causing damage to teeth, bones, kidneys, muscles, nerves, the brain, and immune function. It may also cause genetic damage. Even the Centers for Disease Control and Prevention is now worried that Americans are getting too much fluoride. I've always been puzzled by the warning on children's toothpaste that says, "Keep out of reach of children under 6 years of age. If more than used for brushing is accidentally swallowed, get medical help or contact a Poison Control Center right away." Why? Apparently, there's enough fluoride in that toothpaste tube to severely harm a child. Obviously, one of the best ways to reduce your exposure is to use organic toothpastes that do not contain it.

- Switch to organic lawn and garden products. You can reduce your exposure to harmful garden chemicals by using organic fertilizers. A company called Scotts makes Miracle-Gro Organic Choice, a product line that includes not just fertilizer but also potting and garden soil. The main ingredients are sphagnum peat moss, bark, and a natural source of manure.
- Use earth-friendly cleaning and laundry products. There's a whole new generation of products available these days, made without toxic petrochemicals, that work as well as their chemical counterparts. These safer products are biodegradable, meaning they break down easily in water, and are made with plant-based detergents, botanicals, and natural enzymes. You can also mix up your own cleaners. For example, to clean windows and other glass, mix a gallon of water with 1 cup of white vinegar, apply with a cloth or spray bottle, and dry with a clean cloth. Or try this drain cleaner: Pour $1/2$ cup of baking soda and $1/2$ cup of vinegar down the drain. Let stand for about 10 minutes, then flush with $1/2$ gallon of boiling water.
- Make your own insecticides. Most standard insecticides are synthetic chemicals that kill bugs because they are neurotoxic, meaning they damage the nervous systems of the insects and kill them. But they can damage your nervous system as well. Insecticides have also been linked to Parkinson's disease and numerous other medical problems. Homemade insecticides are a healthier alternative to these potentially dangerous commercial products. Some examples: Talcum powder or chalk is an effective barrier against ants when placed along their line of entry. Red chili powder will repel them, too. Make a paste by mixing the powder with a little water, then apply it to the area where ants are coming in and going out. A dish containing equal parts sugar and baking soda will attract roaches, and the baking soda is deadly to them. Chopped bay leaves and cucumber skins can repel roaches as well. To make an excellent natural insecticide for indoor and outdoor plants, mix 2 tablespoons of liquid soap with 1 quart of water and spray on the leaves.

UP NEXT

In sports, athletic ability is supposed to fade after the age of 30, with the body and mind scheming to make us slower, weaker, and less competitive. But today, the bar has been raised for athletes. Many men and women are active in sports at an advanced age; I'm just one of them. Michael Jordan's well-publicized comeback was underpinned by a workout program designed to reawaken the muscle activity he had as a player and to restore his conditioning so he wouldn't get tired during games. In refusing to age, George Foreman won a heavyweight title in 1994 at age 45. Wayne Gretzky is an enormously gifted athlete, but added to his gift was a weight-training program that helped him survive in his world of crosschecks, bodychecks, and hipchecks as he got older.

Most Americans want to look young and healthy. Some do it with liposuction, plastic surgery, wrinkle creams, or hairpieces. Others do it the way some of our most accomplished (and older!) athletes do it: with the best fountain of youth of all—exercise. That's where we're headed next.

Chapter 6

Step 5:
BUILD THE FITNESS
TO FUNCTION

I can't imagine not being active.
I would do that only by default.

People often say that I'm ahead of trends when it comes to nutrition and fitness. Maybe there's some truth to that; I don't know. I have been going to homeopathic doctors for more than 20 years, and I started doing Pilates in 1989, so I have been ahead of the curve a little bit, I guess.

I do know, however, that I've been doing "functional fitness" and "functional exercise" for more than 2 decades, and today these terms are the latest buzzwords you hear at the gym! Basically, they refer to building a body capable of performing real-life activities, whether that means playing your sport, having the strength to hold a toddler in one arm, carrying luggage without throwing your back out, or being able to keep your balance when a rug slips from under your feet. It also means building a body that defies the normal processes of physical aging. You can look and feel youthful, even as you get older.

Functional exercises, which mimic everyday life to some degree, improve balance, enhance posture, boost stamina, and strengthen your body's core muscles in the torso so you'll be in better shape to tackle your daily activities easily and more safely. They teach the muscles to work in harmony rather than isolating them to work solo, so your body has better stability, balance, and muscle control. Functional training includes enough cardiovascular and strength training to maintain a healthy body. It does not mean becoming a bodybuilder or a marathon runner, but instead staying fit and healthy so your body can handle a wide range of physical challenges. When you're functionally fit, you can lead a life free of strain, injury, and physical restrictions related to your lifestyle; you can count on your body to perform for you, however athletic or nonathletic you may be.

You also have the physical and mental energy to complete your daily tasks at 100 percent effort without feeling run-down at the end of the day or getting mentally tired. I remember one time I had a really hard, intense workout with Billie Jean King. We were getting down to the basics, working on a lot of technical stuff, and breaking everything down. Later that day, I had to set up a new fax machine for my office. I started studying the directions, reading them over and over again, yet I couldn't make head nor tails of them. They weren't complicated; they weren't even written in legalese (which you can't understand on a good day!). I spent 20 minutes trying to comprehend them before I finally gave up. It was hopeless because I was just so tired.

The next morning, I tried again and was able to get the fax machine up and running in a few minutes. The problem hadn't been that my brain wasn't working; I just didn't have the alertness and self-control to concentrate and focus because I was mentally and physically exhausted from that workout. When you're functionally fit, your mind and body don't hold you back from finishing a task, whatever it is. It's natural to be tired at the end of the day, but you shouldn't be so exhausted that you can't think.

It's no accident that chess players work out to maintain the functional fitness they need. You might think they'd be fat because they just sit at a table, but the best chess players train physically so they can play the best chess of their lives. The mind-body connection is so profound that it's impossible to maintain a high level of concentration for several hours if your physical body is ready to give out in 1 hour. You've got to be physically tough if you expect to be mentally tough.

So what's an example of a functional exercise? Think of the squat. When you do it in the conventional manner on a stable surface, you work your thighs and butt. But if you do it while standing on an unstable surface, such as a balance dome, or do a one-legged squat, your body has to work harder. You'll get in shape faster and build balance, control, and stability at the same time.

The squat is also an example of a functional "closed kinetic chain" exercise. This generally means that at least one limb of the ones being exercised is in a fixed position, in constant contact with the surface (such as a pedal, a platform, or the ground), and cannot move, as opposed to an "open kinetic chain" exercise such as an arm curl, in which the hands are not in contact with the surface.

Why is that significant? Your body is put together in a series of kinetic (moving) links or chains that operate in sequence. This kinetic chain produces power and control in sports as well as in many daily activities. Serving a tennis ball, for example, doesn't involve just the arms. The movement begins at your feet, continues up your knees and legs, uses the hips, and involves rotation of the shoulders, arms, and finally the wrist to hit the ball. All body parts move in a fluid series.

Good performance stems from muscles working together rather than from isolated joint movements—which is why closed kinetic chain exercises are so effective for building functional fitness. They develop more muscles, particularly in patterns similar to those used in sports and daily activities, and involve complex movements that cross multiple joints. Plus, they require more balance and stability than open kinetic chain exercises.

I'm always learning which workout I need to get myself in shape, but whatever I do, I train so that I can stay functionally fit—for athletics and for my life. Like a race car driver who takes care of his racing car, I try to treat my body as the temple that it is. After all, it is my livelihood. If I'm good to my body, it will be good to me.

You'll find my favorite functional exercises in Chapter 9, and I'll help you build your own program around them. The exercises I do will challenge you, no matter what your age or current physical shape. Mine isn't a rigorous, body-jarring program, either. In fact, I think you'll like the principles behind this "trend"—and you'll get to like the new you once you incorporate it into your life.

DEVELOP POSTURE AWARENESS

From my earliest schooldays, I had to sit up straight on old wooden benches, and the teachers made us keep our hands behind our backs on the theory that it would improve our posture. They were very rigid about our posture. We had to raise our hands up very straight and high when we had something to say, and we were supposed to raise only our index and middle fingers. Sometimes I would lean straight back against the back of my bench and keep my arm up all the time because I usually knew the answers. Maybe that built up my muscles for my serve!

Looking back, I'm glad they were strict about posture because it gave me enough strength and control to hold my body in proper alignment whether I'm sitting, standing, or moving. If you have inadequate posture in any way, such as a swayback or hunchback, this can create a muscular imbalance and physical stress. Slouching, in particular, as so many of us

BENEFITS OF FUNCTIONAL TRAINING

- Improves posture
- Enhances body control
- Improves balance
- Reduces risk of injury
- Improves sports performance
- Has a positive effect on spinal health
- Tones and strengthens muscles
- Improves speed, agility, and mobility
- Enhances flexibility

do over our computers and desks, can compress internal organs and stress the neck, shoulders, and lower back.

As an athlete, one of the things you're taught to understand is the importance of a "neutral spine." This means aligning your spine into its natural S-shape, in which your body is able to function from its strongest, most balanced position. When you're in this neutral position, stress to your joints, muscles, spine, and other parts of your body is minimized, and you're less likely to hurt yourself. You can move more efficiently when playing sports or exercising. One thing you can say about the greatest athletes is that they make it look easy, and the reason is that they are in neutral most of the time.

If you have trouble working from a neutral posture, it's probably because you have some muscular imbalances. Imagine trying to balance a load of books, and one of the books is sticking out too far. The load is unstable. Similarly, when you're not working from neutral alignment, your body is unstable. This can make certain movements difficult and your body more injury prone.

If you don't move well, you look old, no matter how good your body, hair, clothes, or makeup look. Poor posture has an aging effect, whereas good posture is attractive and gives you a special presence and air of confidence when you walk through a room.

FOLLOWING THROUGH

- You can correct posture problems and learn how to maintain a neutral spine with some simple exercises to strengthen the affected

muscles and compensate for the misalignment of your spine. Some effective posture exercises are included in Chapter 9; they'll help you improve your shoulder position if you tend to slouch and the exaggeration of your spine if you're prone to a swayback.

- In addition to these exercises, try to stay aware of your posture while sitting and standing. When sitting, lift your head and keep your eyes forward. Pull your chin in slightly so your head and neck are lined up. Lift your chest and pull your shoulders back so you don't slouch.
- When you're standing, try to keep your hips, knees, and heels stacked in alignment, with your body weight centered over your feet and your spine in an erect, neutral position.

DEVELOP CORE STRENGTH

Being a good athlete has demanded that I have a strong, stable "core." This refers to all the muscles of your torso and pelvis—the area of your body, including your abdominal muscles, that supports your spine. Like the trunk of a tree supporting its branches, these muscles also help stabilize your body as it moves. For tennis, having a strong core has helped me be able to change direction quickly and generate more force and speed on my strokes.

The biggest benefit of core training, though, is that it develops functional fitness. That's because your core comes into play just about every time you move. When your core is strong, it improves control, balance, and performance while helping prevent injury. Your core is a powerful foundation for your legs and arms, too—which means you can put more force be-hind each step and run more efficiently. When you exercise your core, you also tone your abs, keep your lower back strong, and improve your posture.

FOLLOWING THROUGH

- Begin to strengthen your core with the simple exercises I've included in Chapter 9.
- To vary the types of resistance and reduce boredom, use exercise tubing, free weights, and your own body weight to challenge your core muscles uniquely.
- Concentrate on maintaining proper posture and balance while performing core exercises.
- Progress to exercising on unstable surfaces, such as a balance board, a foam roller, or a device called an Xerdisc, to improve your stability and balance. My exercises include these pieces of equipment.
- Be sure to include stretching exercises to improve flexibility and range of motion in your trunk and hips. You'll find some great stretches in Chapter 9.

BUILD YOUR OVERALL STRENGTH

It's funny how I used to be the skinniest, scrawniest little player in the Czech Republic, all ears and feet and competing against girls a head taller than me, and now I'm pretty muscular. Nature gave me some of those muscles, but others I found in the gym one day, right next to the weight machines. It's like the advertisement says: I got my muscles the old-fashioned way. I earned them.

It was in 1981 that I began to spend more time on exercise machines. One day I'd work on my triceps, biceps, and legs; the next, my chest, shoulders, and back. I also learned how to break down my tennis strokes into functional workouts using cable machines and dumbbells.

These days, I don't have as much strength as I used to because it decreases with age. In fact, women over 25 can lose up to half a pound of muscle mass per year. I can get stronger, but I don't need to hit the weight room the way I used to. I've learned that you don't necessarily need dumbbells, barbells, and machines to build strength. In fact, to get functionally fit, you may want to forget weights at first and learn how to lift and control your own body weight instead. Sure, you may be able to get on a leg-press machine and press 180 or 200 pounds, but you may not be able to do a one-legged squat without tipping over because you don't have the strength of all your muscles working in sync.

Weight machines let us progress to lifting big amounts of weight in all kinds of directions, but that isn't how we normally move in real life. And they don't help build balance. We are always fighting to stay in balance—and I'm talking about physical stuff here (for mental help, that would be another book)—getting in and out of a car, reaching back in your car to get something out of the backseat or comfort a crying child, reaching to get something off a high shelf, or bending over to pick up a child or, in my case, a dog. All of these movements require balance.

A good first step in developing strength is to teach your body to control, lift, and balance its own body weight. Later, I've included some simple movements you can try. What's more, there are inexpensive exercise "toys" you can use at home to build strength and condition your body. Some of the best ones are listed in "10 Toys for Exercise Fun at Home" on page 80. Keep in mind, though, that equipment and exercise toys are secondary. What's most important is the consistent effort you put forth that will get the results you want.

Once you feel your body becoming stronger, by all means, consider weight training. For women in particular, weight training can build bone density in addition to strength, and research shows that the more weight women lift, the more bone they build. It isn't a coincidence that when I had my bone density tested, I was told that my numbers were equivalent to those of a 30-year-old. Since in this country, we no longer need to carry water or wood miles and miles to our homes, we need to do exercises to get the bone-building effects of the physical activity that our grandmothers did naturally in their day-to-day tasks.

Also, if you weight train, your metabolism will run higher and keep burning more calories for as long as 2 hours after your workout. All forms of strength training can increase your independent-function skills if you're an older adult and therefore may help you stay fit and active well into your golden years.

FOLLOWING THROUGH

- To strengthen your body, you can use free weights (dumbbells and barbells), cables, exercise machines, exercise tubing, weighted bars, or your own body weight. When you vary the equipment you use, your workouts won't get stale, and you'll be more psyched up to train.

- Try to work on muscle strengthening a minimum of 2 nonconsecutive days a week. If you're not well conditioned, do one exercise per muscle group (2 or 3 sets of 8 to 12 repetitions). If you're more conditioned, do two or three exercises per muscle group (2 or 3 sets of 8 to 12 repetitions). A twice-weekly strength-training program is doable for most busy people, and you'll achieve good results that can be maintained over time.

- When building strength, be sure to include at least one exercise for each major muscle group: thighs, chest, back, shoulders, arms, abdominals, and calves.

- Each time you work out, do a little more than before—add a few repetitions or another set of repetitions or use a little more weight if you feel up to it. Increasing your effort and working your way up in poundage are what build strength.

- Breathe naturally as you work out; never hold your breath.

REGENERATE

If your muscles and joints ever feel stiff and inflexible, this can be a result of stress, inactivity, overtraining, injury, or degeneration due to aging. Because I'm in my forties, one of my main concerns is flexibility, which we tend to lose with age. Stretching has become very important to me, so I stretch before and after each

10 TOYS FOR EXERCISE FUN AT HOME

EXERCISE TOY	HOW IT WORKS
Balance board	This tool twists and torques with your body's movements for a highly effective total-body workout, including core development. You can use it for standing, lying, and stepping and for functional upper-body movements.
Balancing equipment	Developing good balance is key to performing daily activities and maintaining a functional and independent lifestyle. You can build balance and stability with any number of products, including balance pads, wobble boards, and half-round balance domes.
Dumbbells	These are basic tools you can use to start conditioning your body, and there are literally hundreds of exercises you can do with them. Have a set of dumbbells ranging from 5 to 20 pounds on hand so you can gradually increase your poundage in various exercises to build your strength and remake yourself physically.
Exercise stick	This is a specially designed bar that helps stretch the back, shoulders, torso, and arms.
Exercise tubing	Exercise tubing, or an exercise band, is a length of flexible, stretchable rubber with handles on the ends for comfort and easy use. You can use it to work virtually any muscle group. It comes in several strengths for different levels of difficulty, determined by the elasticity and the color of the band. Some bands come with door anchors and clips so you can attach them to doorjambs in order to perform exercises. Some of the best functional exercises can be done with exercise tubing. Depending on the exercise, tubing provides balance and stability training.
Foam roller	The foam roller is an effective balance and alignment tool for developing core stabilization, lower-body balance, and stamina and for regenerating muscles and soft tissue as part of a total fitness program.
Jump rope	This well-known piece of aerobic equipment helps build cardiovascular fitness, condition your muscles, and burn calories.
Medicine ball	Exercising with a medicine ball helps you execute movements that require shifting, bending, rotating, and balance, all of which are important in athletics and in life. Throwing a medicine ball in certain exercises also helps you build speed, power, strength, flexibility, better coordination, stability, and joint integrity.
Stability ball	The stability ball is useful for developing balance, core strength, and basic body strength. Stabilizing exercises done on the ball also help improve joint function.
Weighted bar	This functional training tool comes in a variety of weights and is ideal for developing strength, balance and alignment, core strength, and flexibility.

workout. Sometimes that might be three times a day. I don't particularly like it, but I know how much it helps me recover and regenerate from tough matches or workouts and gets me ready to go the next day. If you don't stretch, you can have a great day or two, but then on the third day, you can't seem to find the court, no matter what. It's much more difficult to recover physically if you don't have a good stretching program in place.

One of the ways I've found to maximize my recovery time is to stretch using a foam roller, which you can buy for less than $20. Foam roller stretches work by freeing up the fascia, the soft tissue that encases your muscles, nerves, and blood vessels. The fascia can become restricted because of injury, inflexibility, or overuse, and this causes tight muscles, muscle soreness, and poor range of motion. Using special exercises with the foam roller, you can massage away these restrictions. You simply roll an area of your body along the roller, breaking down tight areas and improving bloodflow to your muscles.

When I first started using the foam roller, parts of my body hurt so badly that I could put barely any pressure on them, especially in an area called the iliotibial (IT) band, a tough group of fibers that run along the outside of the thigh. Now I can put all my weight on the roller, and it feels very soothing on my body. My IT band is looser than it has been in ages, as is the rest of my body. Sometimes I feel like cookie dough being rolled out when I use the roller, and it feels good.

In Chapter 9, I demonstrate how to use a foam roller with a series of exercises that will help improve your flexibility and function, manage muscle soreness, improve range of motion, and reduce injuries.

FOLLOWING THROUGH

- Stretch a warm muscle, never a cold one. Begin your workout with a 5- to 10-minute warmup on some cardiovascular equipment, such as a stationary bicycle, or do some walking. This will increase your body temperature and warm up your muscles.
- Stretch before and after exercise.
- Don't bounce while you stretch. Bouncing invites your muscles to tighten up in order to protect themselves. Ease into your stretch with moves that are slow and controlled. Stretch to a point of tension but never pain.
- Keep breathing. Don't hold your breath while stretching; instead, keep your breathing even and consistent. This will help relax your body. With each exhalation, you can stretch farther.
- Hold each stretch for 10 to 20 seconds and stretch each muscle group two or three times.

REMAKE YOUR BODY

Maybe you're thinking, "Okay, functional exercises will improve the quality of my everyday life, but will they change the way my body looks?"

Absolutely. With functional training, you work all your muscle groups, large and small, with a very concentrated effort, so you're definitely going to see changes in your shape. You recruit many different muscle groups, so you'll burn calories and fat more efficiently.

If you're not looking in too many mirrors these days, if you can't fit into your clothes, or if you're feeling depressed about your appearance, I've got several exercises in Chapter 9 that will sculpt and shape your body where it needs it the most.

FOLLOWING THROUGH

- Individualize your program based on which body parts you want to reshape. If your legs need more muscle definition, for example, you might add an extra leg exercise or two to your routine, plus do some running or cycling.

- When designing your routine, be sure to do exercises that work all major muscle groups in addition to those you want to target for extra shaping. Working certain muscle groups at the expense of others can lead to muscle imbalances and possible injury.
- If you don't see the desired results after 4 to 6 weeks, change your routine. Introduce new exercises into your workout.
- Consult a qualified personal trainer to help you put together a routine that will help you meet your body-shaping goals.

TUNE UP YOUR CARDIOVASCULAR SYSTEM

Just as the muscles of your body need to be strengthened, your heart muscle needs to be strengthened. Cardiovascular, or aerobic, exercise trains the heart, lungs, and circulatory system to work more efficiently and enables you to climb a flight of stairs or play your sport without getting out of breath.

There are lots of other benefits, too. Cardio exercise:

- Burns fat and calories.
- Revs up your metabolism.
- Releases endorphins, your body's natural painkillers.
- Increases the concentration of good cholesterol (HDL) in your blood and lowers the concentration of bad cholesterol (LDL).
- Reduces your risk of heart disease, high blood pressure, stroke, type 2 diabetes, and some cancers.
- Stimulates your immune system to ward off illnesses.

Often, though, people have such poor cardiovascular fitness that they can barely walk through a mall without huffing and puffing. Getting regular aerobic exercise—without going overboard—will give you more energy. When you're aerobically fit, your body takes in and uses oxygen to support muscle movement more efficiently, pumps blood faster and more forcefully to produce energy, and increases the diameter and number of capillaries (small blood vessels) for better oxygen delivery and waste removal. Aerobic exercise also pumps more blood to your brain to make you feel more alert and helps you better handle emotional stress.

FOLLOWING THROUGH

- Select cardiovascular exercises based on your present level of conditioning and skill level. For example, you don't want to start running if you've never run before; it's better to start with a walking program.
- Find a cardiovascular activity that you enjoy doing and will want to continue indefinitely.
- Ideally, cardiovascular training should be done a minimum of three to five times a week for 30 to 45 minutes each time. But even twice a week for just 30 minutes will make a difference in how you will feel. Your workout can be as simple as walking or using

a treadmill or stair-stepping machine or as challenging as running several miles a day. Gradually try to increase the intensity of your workout, and keep tabs on how well you're progressing. You can use the Perceived Exertion Scale (see page 206) to help gauge your intensity.

- Start slowly. Before any workout, you want to raise your core temperature by doing a slow jog or fast walk for 5 minutes.
- Cool down afterward with light cardiovascular activity and some stretching exercises.

LESS IS MORE

As an athlete, I always try to push the envelope when it comes to increasing my performance. But like every other hard-training athlete, I tend to overdo things from time to time and succumb to a physical condition known as overtraining. Overtraining happens when you push your body past the point of full recovery for your next workout. When you exercise, you tear down your body to some extent, and it needs sufficient time, rest, and nutrition to recover. If you push too far and too hard before your body is ready to handle the effort, you can cause injury or illness or lapse into a drained and depleted condition. Signs of overtraining include excessive fatigue, insomnia, decreased performance, nagging muscle or joint pain, and more frequent illnesses and upper respiratory infections.

You do not have to train like a world-class athlete to get in great shape, nor do you have to push yourself to the absolute limit to be successful with exercise. I've had friends who sometimes did too much physically, even if a doctor told them not to. Their thinking was that more is better, whereas I have now come to believe in doing less rather than more. Far too many people these days are caught up in this more-is-better exercise philosophy—more weight on the bench press, more situps, more time on the treadmill, a higher level on the stair-stepper while hanging on to the rail for dear life, more aerobics classes. More, more, more.

Overtraining like this is not good for you, just as overeating is not good for you. When you exercise beyond what your body tells you is acceptable, you risk putting it in a state of physical, chemical, and mental imbalance. It's better to err on the side of working out a little less than to work out too much. Even though I advised you earlier to try to push yourself to do a little more in each workout, do so only in moderation and with good form so your body can handle it.

If I have no energy the day after a training session, I know I've completely shot my body. With the right amount of training, you should feel energized by your workouts, not so draggy that you don't want to get out of bed or so sore that you can't lift your arms to brush your teeth.

So how much exercise do you need? When I took woodworking lessons a few years ago, I picked up some unique insight that will help me answer that question. There were about 12 of us in the class, all asking technical questions of our teacher.

"How much angle do you need for a proper dovetail joint?"

"Just enough," replied the teacher.

"How much glue do you need?"

"Just enough."

"How much sanding does it take?"

"Just enough."

And so it went.

My training is "just enough" to give me what I need for what I do. I don't do a huge volume of training, but my workouts are concentrated and very specific and intense. I don't spend a great amount of time working out, but I know everything that I do is very productive.

The keys, really, are balance and variety, without overdoing any one component of training. I could spend more time running a little faster, but it's not necessary because I'd be sacrificing something else. I have to balance my training around the time I spend on the court, on strategy, on technique, on fitness, on my core, or on flexibility. I need all of it to be a complete, functional athlete, but I do all of it in moderation. For you, it's the same: In order to be a healthy, functionally fit adult, you need that balance. You need that variety. You can't concentrate on just one area, such as aerobics, or another area is going to suffer. I know people who are runners. That's all they do—run every single day. You know what? They don't look healthy. They're so gaunt and shriveled up that they remind me of 150-pound raisins.

Your body is always sending messages about what it requires. You want to start listening, because it can keep you in great shape or, more important, it may save your life. You've got to listen to what your body needs for all-around health and fitness. As far as exercise is concerned, maybe now you're con-

centrating on strength, but make sure you are doing enough stretching to keep your muscles long and supple. Maybe you're doing a lot of cardio, but you need to supplement it with work on good balance and core strength. It's all about fine-tuning, paying attention to what works and what doesn't, and then changing accordingly—and doing just enough without overdoing it.

Today's young athletes could benefit from taking the less-is-more approach to sports. From the time I started school, tennis was my sport, but I did other things, too. In the summer, I played soccer and swam in the river. In the winter, I skated on the river, played ice hockey, and went downhill and cross-country skiing. Most of it was for fun, not so much for competition.

I look at some of the kids coming along today, and their lives are all competitive sports. It's no wonder that doctors in pediatric sports medicine feel that they've happened upon a new childhood disease—overuse injuries in kids. The cause is the overaggressive culture of organized youth sports.

According to an article in the *New York Times* in 2005, the injuries doctors are seeing include stress fractures, growth plate disorders, cracked kneecaps, frayed heel tendons, and back injuries. All of these are injuries once seen only in adults.

In the past, kids who were normally active played a lot of different sports, as I did, sometimes all in the same day. That was good for their bodies, so they could develop in balance. Now, though, so many young athletes specialize so early in their lives that they exclude other sports. They end up playing just that one sport year-round, doing the same drills over and over. Their parents and coaches keep them from doing other sports so they don't get hurt, but guess what? They get hurt—badly. Instead of the typical sprained ankle or bruised knee, they have torn Achilles tendons, or they may require knee reconstruction or elbow surgery. Once again, it's all about balance.

I've seen this myself in tennis. The young girls are working harder than we used to, and they're in better shape. But I think in my time, we were better athletes because we played other sports. We weren't as specialized as this generation is. Now it's tennis, tennis, tennis. Today's players are great at hitting the ball, but when they fall, they get hurt because they have no idea how to fall. I played so many different sports all through my life that I learned how to fall without hurting myself. Yes, I still fall on the court, and I might scrape my knee a little bit, but I've never had a serious injury.

FOLLOWING THROUGH

- Take rest periods, such as a day between workouts, to let your body recuperate and re-generate. It gets to be a case of diminishing returns. Doing more and more—without building rest and recovery into your routine—does you less and less good. It's the quality of training that counts, not the quantity.
- Vary your workouts from light to heavy or gradually increase the intensity to a certain level, then back off.
- Fight overtraining with food. Sometimes changes in your diet are needed to meet the demands of increased exercise. You may

have to take in more calories, carbohydrates, or protein.
- Make notes in your journal about your food choices, your exercise schedule, and how you feel physically and emotionally to help you keep track of what's working well and what isn't.

FIND A TRAINING PARTNER

Even though tennis is an individual game—just you and your opponent, sometimes with a crowd watching—I've always liked team sports: passing the puck to somebody in an ice hockey game or kicking the ball to someone in a soccer match. There's camaraderie in it all, with the encouragement from the bench, talking over the game on the way home, and just having fun together during and after the game. There's ful-fillment in being around people you like. When people encourage you and make you feel good, you want to be around them, which is why I prefer training with a workout partner.

Sure, you can work out by yourself, but having a partner helps you get motivated and work harder. You'll probably run faster and farther when you run with a friend than if you run alone, and you will most likely have more fun. You're less likely to cop out and not do it. You have a scheduled commitment with someone, and you don't want to let them down. You want to help them get better. There's a synergy that helps both of you strive for your best.

FOLLOWING THROUGH

- A good place to find a training partner is at your gym. Ask the manager if he knows of

WHAT I'VE LEARNED ABOUT EXERCISE

- Go out there and have fun. That's what exercise should be about, but unfortunately, we have de-funned exercise in this country, making it a chore or an obliga-tion. The more fun I'm having, the better I train.

- Follow an exercise routine in which there is no routine. Whenever something becomes routine, you don't pay attention to it anymore. I rarely do the same routine twice, which keeps me interested and focused.

- Do your exercises right, and you won't have to do as many reps. Correct technique is what makes exercise harder, not necessarily the volume.

- Do your workout first thing in the morning whenever possible so it doesn't get canceled at the end of the day. For a lot of peo-ple, it's always their workouts that get the boot when sched-ules are tight.

- Stay consistent. When you get older, you can't just take a week off and pick up right where you left off. You have to keep at it. I do something every day, even if it's only for a half hour. At my age, frequency is far more important than working out 3 hours on Saturday and doing nothing the rest of the week. Your body is like a sports car. If you run it more often, it runs better. Let it sit for a month, and you've got problems.

- Mix it up by performing many dif-ferent activities. Since, like most tennis players, I have the atten-tion span of the average humming-bird, I've always liked to have great variety in my training. Here are all the things I might do on any given day (although not all at once): basketball, ice hockey, mountain biking, swimming, hik-ing, soccer, softball, running, kick-ing a Hacky Sack, running track, skiing, snowboarding, Pilates, and lots of on-court drills to keep up my speed and agility. The body is lazy. Once it gets used to a pat-tern, it will work just enough— no more, no less—to stay there. To continue getting more fit and in shape, don't let your body be-come complacent. Keep it work-ing and guessing. Stimulate your muscles in fresh ways to shock your body (in a good way) into continued adaptation.

- Keep your mind occupied while working out. Concentrate on other members who might like to have a partner. Or, if you're not a member of a gym, maybe there's a friend or someone in your neighborhood or at work who might like to work out at home with you or go run-ning or biking with you.
  - Join a biking or running club to hook up with a suitable partner.

- Look for a prospective partner who has the same drive and dedication you have and shares most of your training interests, abili-ties, and goals. Make sure your schedules match, too, so you can work out on the same days and at the same times.
  - Try to find a partner who's a little stronger or faster than you are, or at least on the

your breathing, your heart rate, your technique, or your performance. It's like flying a plane. When I was taking flying lessons, the instructors taught me to look everywhere all the time, to scan the horizon without zeroing in on any single thing. So it is with exercise. You can make the workout fun within yourself when you monitor what your body is doing.

- Breathe through your nose, especially when doing cardiovascular exercise. It gets better-quality air into your lungs. It's almost impossible to overdo your workout when you breathe this way. You will feel refreshed when you're done, rather than exhausted. If you feel the need to breathe through your mouth to catch your breath, do it, but in the meantime, slow down until you can breathe through your nose again. That way, you won't wear your body down.

- Make your workout a challenge by setting goals. Keep track of your progress so you can see how far you've come and how close you are to your objectives.

- With all forms of exercise, pick something you like to do. There's no sense in running unless you like to run.

- Do something you're pretty good at or can at least master. If you're all left feet on the dance floor, you probably won't feel successful in an aerobic dance class. Find an activity you can do with confidence. Confidence creates the inner environment to succeed and stay with it.

- Have a plan for when you're going to exercise each week. You'll be much more time efficient. If you don't have a half hour a day or at least an hour three times a week to spend on yourself, you need to reorganize your life. Something's not right. If you don't have any time for yourself, whose life are you living?

- If you're a competitive athlete, be careful what you do in your off-season. You don't want to pull muscles, break bones, or otherwise put yourself out of commission. For example, I didn't start snowboarding until after my retirement from tennis because I was afraid of injuring myself. Fortunately, I have never broken even a fingernail snowboarding.

same level athletically. It is more of a challenge and pushes you to be better than you are. I find that I work out harder when I'm with a partner. I enjoy it more, and I find it more fulfilling because on those days when I'm a little low on energy, when my get-up-and-go has gotten up and gone, I kick in when my partner kicks in. I also love helping my partner get more out of herself or himself.

HOW I LEARNED TO LOVE EXERCISE

I don't mind admitting that there was a time in my life when I didn't like formal exercise. I would go to any length to avoid it. Truthfully, it was a love-hate relationship in that I didn't really like the pain, but I loved what exercise did for me. Can you relate? All that changed during the Team Navratilova years, when I worked out with Nancy Lieberman and hooked up with a coach, and together they devised a series of exercises and drills on and off the court to improve virtually every aspect of my game. They pushed me and kept me going, and I could see and feel the difference in my physical and mental shape. It was hard going, but I knew that it was going to lead somewhere. I began to enjoy exercising. Now I love working out, and I love the way I feel afterward.

You can have the same experience if you're willing to break your habit of inactivity. Each time you work out, you'll be happy that you did it and that you didn't quit or take the easy way out. What have you got to lose? You'll look and feel better. You'll have more energy. You'll feel stronger and more physically fit because you *are* stronger and more fit. Also,

you'll know that you have the power to get out there and make the effort to improve your well-being and quality of life. You will have a concrete reason to move through life with more confidence and self-assurance. Start today—why not?—and expect to notice a big difference in your quality of life within a few weeks. In a month, you will be astonished at how you look as well as how you feel.

If exercising seems like too much work, maybe you need to look at your energy level. That's what we'll do in the next step. A frustrating and unsatisfying part of life is that many of us have only a passing acquaintance with energy and vitality. When you constantly feel drained, lifestyle habits are usually to blame. If you're tired all the time—and tired of feeling that way—don't take it lying down. In the next chapter, we'll talk about how to tweak your nutrition and lifestyle so you'll have loads more energy to live the life you want to live.

CHAPTER 7

STEP 6:

RECHARGE AND ENERGIZE—WHEN YOU'RE TIRED OF BEING TIRED

If your life is to be enjoyed and not endured, then your days must be enjoyed and not endured.

One thing I've noticed about a lot of people—even players on the tour—is that they go around complaining about how tired they are. You see them dragging, and you ask, "How do you feel?" Their automatic response is, "I'm really tired."

Feeling tired all the time should not be a normal state, unless of course you're overexerting yourself physically, not sleeping enough, or not eating properly. I do know what it's like to feel totally spent, unable to enjoy the things you like to do. I was skiing in Aspen on one very beautiful day—the kind that doesn't come along very often. There I was, gliding down the mountain, yet I had to stop after a couple of hours because I was feeling so tired. Practically breathless, I couldn't locate my lungs, and my legs felt like they were going to buckle underneath me.

The problem was my habits at the time. As I mentioned earlier, I had gained weight after I retired from singles competition; I wasn't paying a lot of attention to what I was eating nor was I doing nearly as much physically as I had when I was on tour. I hadn't been working at keeping my body fit, and I was in such an unconditioned state, it was pathetic. My way of living had taken something out of me. That day in Aspen, I told myself, "This is really stupid—if I were in better condition, I could enjoy the whole day." So that's when I started getting my health habits back in order. I didn't like feeling so out of commission.

I'm convinced that a lot of the fatigue I see is because people are tired mentally, they're tired emotionally, and they're sort of industrially tired—in other words, their lives make them tired. If I feel drained, it's usually because I've had a hard workout or I'm not eating the right foods. My life doesn't make me tired. The way I see it, your life should excite you, not drain you.

If you think about it, using the word *drain* to describe your energy level has some basis in truth. Your body is an energy source. In that sense, it is a living battery. When you're low on energy, your body is like a battery with a low charge, with all the "juice" draining out of it. Like a battery, it needs to recharge. When it does, your ability to think clearly, create, function, and feel vital improves greatly.

Feeling tired all the time means that your body's resources are drained—and strained. Fatigue is your body's way of telling you something is wrong. Learn to listen to that message. Right now, stop and take the energy quiz below. It will alert you to whether you may need to consult a physician about your "energy crisis." Low energy is poor health. Ask yourself: Do you barely want to get out of bed, or do you want to jump out, feeling rested and excited to be alive? If you're tired of being tired, you can do something about it because most fatigue is lifestyle related. You don't have to live with constant tiredness.

YOUR ENERGY CONDITION

Feeling tired or run-down all the time will prevent you from living an active, healthy lifestyle. Take stock of your energy level and find out whether you're in an energy crisis. Check the statements that apply to you most of the time.

1. I have periodic bouts of fatigue and tiredness.
2. Within the past year, I have experienced a major life stressor—a divorce, death of a loved one, a job change, a move to a new location, financial problems, etc.
3. I have trouble getting a good night's sleep.
4. My fatigue came on suddenly or followed a severe flu-like illness.
5. I get tired easily.
6. I often feel too tired for sex.
7. I'm being treated for a thyroid condition but still experience fatigue.
8. I feel depressed at times.
9. I feel too run-down to exercise.
10. I feel like taking naps most days of the week.

What Your Responses May Mean

If you checked three or more of these statements, chances are you're experiencing fatigue that needs to be addressed with some of the strategies I'll talk about here. Please note:

Questions 2, 4, 7, and 8 may signal a medical or psychological problem underlying your fatigue. Some of these are listed in "Medical Causes of Fatigue" on page 102. Talk to your doctor as soon as you can.

CHECK YOUR PLATE

After I started avoiding processed foods and products that contain additives in favor of natural organic foods and juices, I noticed a near-immediate boost in my energy levels. I didn't really know why, except for the fact that processed and fake foods harbor toxins that are a form of hidden stress on the body. Before I made the switch, I was ingesting toxins that were draining my energy. Those foods are also devoid of vitamins and minerals, whereas natural foods are loaded with these energy-giving nutrients. The body needs nutrients such as iron to deliver oxygen to working muscles, B vitamins to break down food for energy, magnesium to convert food into energy, and zinc to help repair muscle cells. When your body is short on nutrients like those, you can experience fatigue. Changing my diet by making healthier, more nourishing choices certainly revived my energy levels.

A medical journal ran an article a few years ago that fascinated me. It reported on a group of scientists who studied 26 people with fibromyalgia, which causes widespread pain in the body, often accompanied by fatigue, insomnia, headaches, depression, and anxiety. The people in the study were told to eat mostly a raw vegetarian diet that included fresh fruit, salads, raw vegetables, carrot juice, wheatgrass,

nuts, seeds, whole grain foods, flaxseed oil, and extra-virgin olive oil. They were asked to avoid alcohol, caffeine, dairy foods, meat, eggs, and foods containing refined sugar, corn syrup, hydrogenated oil, and refined flour.

What happened toward the end of the experiment was pretty amazing. The new diet produced a dramatic improvement in all of the fibromyalgia symptoms, particularly fatigue and disrupted sleep patterns. Pretty remarkable, I think. This all goes to show that a mostly vegetable-based diet, with plenty of raw foods, can be a healing style of life. If it can manage or even reverse fibromyalgia symptoms so well, just imagine what it can do if you're not having any physical problems! Your energy levels just might go through the roof.

I can relate to that study because over the years, I've learned to identify specific foods that sap my energy. Dairy products are one. Every once in a while, I'll treat myself to a milkshake, usually when I'm in Aspen, where there's a restaurant that makes great milkshakes with premium ice cream, served in huge containers. If I drink the whole thing—which I confess I usually do—my day is done. There is nothing to do afterward except sleep. That's how I feel anytime I eat dairy products: They just put me to sleep. I try to avoid them, and I feel so much better when I do. As for calcium, I get mine from tofu, almond milk, and calcium-rich veggies such as broccoli and greens.

If you follow a more natural-foods style of eating, you should notice improvements in your energy level and other aspects of your health. A living example of what I'm talking about is one of my financial advisors, whom I'll call

John. He's a great guy by most people's standards, and decidedly a computer geek. He spends so much time at the computer that his wife is starting to worry that one of these days, she's going to kiss the computer goodnight, thinking it's the back of her husband's head.

She often complained that John was slower than a turtle and very hard to motivate. I once overheard her challenge him, in loving frustration, to a race with one of their pet turtles, named Achilles. It humorously went like this: "John, you are so slow that I could draw a finish line up the street. You could go and start walking toward it while I went into the house to get Achilles, brought him out, and pointed him toward the line. I bet I could watch him not only pass you but get there a day ahead of you!"

I guess John one day decided that his wife might have a point about his sluggish behavior. He also realized that he couldn't continue feeling so exhausted during the middle of the day because it was affecting his performance. At about the same time, he peaked at 230 pounds. He is 6 feet 5 inches tall, but unfortunately, the excess weight resided right smack in the middle of his body, at his waist. Tummy fat is a bad-news risk factor for heart disease, and John knew it. He wanted to make a real change in his life, not a temporary one.

One evening during dinner, he asked me about my eating habits. We talked about foods I ate as a child, young adult, and athlete. He began to tell me about books he had started to read on the subject simply because he wanted to get in better shape.

John then tried to cleanse his body through fasting—something I do not endorse. I believe it is unrealistic, too much of a shock for the body, and frankly unnecessary. After 2 days, the fast gave him a severe headache, and he became even more tired and sluggish.

His wife asked me to step in and help. I suggested that John make just one change each week by taking something out and substituting something else that he had not tried before. I also asked him to deliberately but gradually reduce his intake of sugar and processed foods, especially breads. He didn't need to cut out these foods altogether, just eat less of them over the course of the week.

The first week, he began enjoying fresh juice for breakfast and had a normal lunch and a normal dinner. Then I suggested he try a smoothie for breakfast. A month later, he had incorporated juicing, smoothies, fruits, and vegetables into his eating habits.

By making a few gradual changes to his diet, John scaled down to 173 pounds of lean body mass. He no longer craves sugar, doesn't eat dairy products, and is careful about how much bread and pasta he eats. His energy level has increased dramatically, so much so that today, he is considering having a go at competitive running.

Over the years, I've learned what works for me, and I don't want to lecture you or say that you have to do everything I do. But I'd like to strongly encourage you to give your body energy-boosting foods like fresh fruits, vegetables, and whole grains and limit energy-draining foods like fatty meats and dairy products, refined sugar, and processed foods. You don't have to do this radically, either—just gradually. For some people, that may mean a month; for others, a whole year. Permanent, positive change takes time to occur, but it will happen as long as you're patient with yourself. Realize that you'll have good days and bad days, but what's important is that you're doing your best to choose foods that make you feel as good as you are able to feel.

FOLLOWING THROUGH

- Eat well—and often. For sustained energy levels throughout the day, eat smaller, more frequent meals (i.e., six meals of approximately 300 to 450 calories each) of pure, wholesome foods like whole grains, fruits, vegetables, and lean protein, such as white-meat poultry or fish.

- Put more raw foods and fresh juices into the mix. For fatigue, natural health experts recommend a diet that includes 50 percent raw foods and fresh juices, all from fruits and vegetables. These foods provide nutrients that renew your energy and make you feel rejuvenated.

- Here's something to try. It comes from my own experience of listening to my body after making some of the choices I've made, either when I've been kind to my health or when I've slid backward. First, think about how you feel the day after making an unhealthy choice—like bingeing on a cheeseburger, fries, and three beers washed down with a shot of tequila. Write about it in your journal. Then, a few days later, have a light, healthy meal, such as a salad and fresh fruit for dessert. Drink a lot of water with it. Pay attention to how you feel the next day and

compare the two experiences. Which way would you rather feel—sluggish or fantastic?

- Steer clear of chocolate, soft drinks, and highly processed foods. These rob your body of magnesium, which can lead to fatigue.

- Be aware of *when* you eat. For most of us, dinner should not be the largest meal of the day. Digesting a big meal may keep you awake, and sleep deprivation is a cause of fatigue. What I like to do is have my biggest meal at noon and eat a light dinner. If you do have a big dinner, try to schedule it early in the evening, say 6:00 p.m., rather than later, when it's close to bedtime.

- Talk to your doctor about the possibility of a food allergy. A lot of people are allergic to common foods such as wheat and dairy products, and the reaction causes fatigue. When they eliminate those foods, they feel less sluggish and less tired. Why is this? Reactions to certain foods cause the release of histamine, a chemical involved in immune response, into the bloodstream. While histamine produces "typical" allergic reactions like sneezing and itchy or burning eyes, it can also cause moodiness and fatigue. If you think you may be sensitive to a certain food, take it out of your diet and then reintroduce it over a period of time. If a food allergy is part of your fatigue problem, you should notice a difference in your energy level several days later.

- Drink plenty of pure water every single day. Dehydration is a hidden source of fatigue. Try drinking 8 ounces of water every 2 to 3 hours during the day, for a total of eight glasses daily. Among other duties, water helps flush toxins from your body that may be making you feel sluggish.

■ Stay mindful of what you need to keep your body in top-notch condition wherever you go. When I travel, for example, I often take my own food on flights. At speaking engagements or photo shoots, I ask for fruits and vegetables (for juicing) in advance. I rarely feel tired when I focus on healthy eating.

REFUEL FOR AN ENERGY EDGE

You burn off energy—in the form of nutrients—when you exercise. Unless you replace those nutrients, namely carbohydrates and protein, you won't help your energy levels, your performance, or your game very much. In fact, you'll invite fatigue. What I've learned to do after a workout or match is replenish my system by eating a little protein and some carbs as a post-exercise snack. When you work out or train for competition, carbohydrates (stored in the muscles as glycogen) supply most of the fuel your body burns for energy, so you have to restock what has been depleted. Unless you do, your body will start burning muscle, and that will tax your energy and drive. Nutritionally fueling your muscles following exercise is what athletes call recovery. Good recovery keeps your body energized.

Carbohydrates are important in another respect: They break down into glucose, which is the major fuel for immune cells. Low blood glucose also triggers the release of stress hormones that suppress immune function, so a drop in blood sugar during and after prolonged, intensive exercise can reduce immunity. If viruses and bacteria gain a foothold during this window of opportunity following hard exercise (3 to 72 hours), you are more susceptible to getting sick. True fitness means being able to resist illness and injury, having the most energy, and looking your best. The solution is to prevent low blood sugar by eating a diet plentiful in carbs and refueling with carbs after workouts.

Focus your post-exercise snacks on wholesome carbohydrates that are digested and absorbed rapidly. They replenish muscle glycogen more readily. Here are some examples of carbs that do the job.

Fresh fruit and vegetable juices

Fresh fruit, such as bananas

Smoothies

Sports drinks, such as Gatorade

Meal-replacement beverages or bars as a source of carbs *and* protein

Raisins

Multigrain bagel

Potato or sweet potato

Corn

Having some protein is important, too. The combination of protein and carbs speeds up the manufacture of new glycogen; it also elevates levels of key hormones in your body that are involved in muscle repair and growth. Here are some good options for refueling with protein.

Tofu

Edamame (steamed soybeans)

Soy milk

Yogurt

Lean chicken or fish

Egg whites

Athletes and exercisers who take recovery nutrition seriously balance their post-exercise snacks in a ratio of 4 parts carbohydrate to 1 part protein. So if you eat 100 grams of carbohydrate after exercising, you should have 25 grams of protein along with it. Another way to figure it is if you eat a cup of chopped fresh fruit, you can top if off with $1/4$ cup of yogurt or soy milk. Some experts believe that eating carbs and protein in this ratio is the most efficient way to replenish your muscles so they can repair and rebuild.

Carbohydrates and protein aren't the only nutrients that need to be replaced. After exercising, it's important to replace the fluids lost through sweating. Drinking eight to ten 8-ounce glasses of water every day is a good practice. What's more, the older you get, the less sensitive your thirst mechanism becomes, so you may need fluids but not feel thirsty. Rehydration is a top nutritional priority after you've exercised.

FOLLOWING THROUGH

- Eat or drink foods (i.e., juices or smoothies) containing carbohydrates in the first 15 minutes after your workout. This time frame promotes the most rapid refueling since the enzymes that make glycogen are at their peak activity then.
- Don't forget protein to enhance recovery. You can accelerate the rate at which your muscles store glycogen as well as speed up the recov-

ery and repair of muscle tissue by eating some protein in combination with carbohydrates following your workout. Just make sure carbohydrates are the foundation of your meal or snack, and protein is the accompaniment.

- Try these refueling combos (they're my favorites): 1 scrambled egg white and half a multigrain bagel; 1 medium banana and $1/2$ cup cottage cheese; 1 small whole wheat pita and 2 tablespoons hummus with a glass of soy milk; a fruit smoothie made with yogurt or soy milk and fruit; fresh vegetable or fruit juice with four whole wheat crackers.

GET QUALITY SLEEP

There have been days when I've run out of strength and I didn't have as much energy as I would have liked, and I know one reason is lack of sleep. Sleep troubles are certainly a huge cause of fatigue. It's essential to get a good night's sleep if you want to be at your sharpest. Sleep deprivation impairs your judgment, reaction time, and other functions. It can also lower your immunity and bring on premature aging. Getting less sleep than you need creates a sleep debt in your body, like being overdrawn at the bank. Before long, your body will demand that the debt be repaid.

What I've learned to do is not fight my body. If I feel tired and sleepy, I go to bed. I like to get about 8 hours of sleep a night—a lot less than that, and I'm groggy the next day.

Some people have said that I'm a night owl, and I used to think so, too. But being a night person had more to do with my tennis lifestyle than with anything else. My matches were usually played in the evenings, so I had to be wide-awake at night. While on the road playing tournaments, I would sleep right through breakfast and normally get up around noon. It usually takes about 4 hours after waking for your physical energy to kick in at 100 percent for a match. I played the majority of my matches at night, so I had to be wide-awake. The first match was typically played at about 6:00 p.m., the second at 7:30, and the last at 9:30, sometimes later. I'd usually get to bed around 2:00 a.m., thus the late start to the day. I always thought I was a night owl, but once I stopped playing in 1994, I found myself going to sleep between 10:00 and 11:00 and waking up at the crack of dawn. Being a night owl was completely a by-product of my lifestyle and not my body's natural choice.

I like to wake up on my own, too; I hate to set an alarm unless I have to catch an early flight or go to an early appointment. But most of us set an alarm every day. It's better—if you can manage it—to wake up with the sun. Sunlight helps your body's biological clock reset itself each day.

Sometimes it's hard to control the time you go to sleep and the time you get up. Most sleep experts will tell you that consistent bedtimes and wake-up times, even on weekends, will improve your sleep and help you feel refreshed every morning.

Fortunately, I've had very few sleepless nights. Jet lag used to mess with my sleep, but I've learned how to conquer it. Today, if I have to be on a plane for several hours, I make the best of it. It's my time. I don't have to answer to anybody, and I can begin to relax. I usually read a book or watch a movie. I drink a lot of water to fight the dehydration (which leads to fatigue) caused by the dry air in the plane. I cut back on how much protein I eat, because protein can keep you awake, and eat more carbs, which have a naturally tranquilizing effect on the body. While I'm on the plane, I synchronize my watch to match the time zone at my destination. This is a mental trick you can play to reset your body clock so you can adapt to the new time zone more easily.

On those rare occasions when I can't get to sleep, I don't just lie in bed tossing and turning and worrying about it. The anxiety of not being able to sleep only makes matters worse. I turn the light on and do something else, such as read or listen to music. Or I meditate and do some deep breathing until my body feels like drifting off to sleep. This works like a charm.

One of the most important ways to get a good night's sleep is to eliminate the "sleep robbers." One of the reasons that I'm a pretty sound sleeper is that I don't drink much coffee or alcohol, nor do I smoke. Coffee, alcohol, and nicotine are sleep robbers—just what the doctor did not order for someone with sleep problems.

As everyone knows, coffee is full of caffeine, as are many teas, chocolate, some soft drinks, and certain over-the-counter medications. Caffeine is a stimulant, which means it has a wake-up effect, and heavy use of coffee—about four cups daily—can cause sleep problems. But even a small amount of coffee early in the day can keep you from falling asleep 10 to 12 hours later, since caffeine stays in the body for roughly 20 hours. I like the taste of coffee but hate its effect on me. If I have a cup, it gives me a kick at first, but an hour later, my energy level comes crashing down. I usually drink decaf, if I drink coffee at all. You might try to cut back on your intake of caffeinated beverages, at least in the afternoon. If you start sleeping better, you've pinpointed the problem.

Alcohol is lethal to good sleep, too. It keeps you in the lighter stages of sleep so you never really achieve restful, restorative sleep. You'll feel lethargic the next day, with little energy or enthusiasm for exercise or recreation. Personally, I've never been much of a drinker, nor have I ever gotten drunk. I guess I'm too much of a control freak to just lose it to alcohol. As soon as I start feeling that way, I stop drinking. Having two beers is my idea of "falling off the wagon." Alcohol certainly doesn't help your body if you're trying to take off excess weight, either. In fact, it slows down your metabolism and is quickly converted to body fat.

What a lot of smokers don't realize is that nicotine, like caffeine, is a stimulant that makes it hard to fall asleep and contributes to problems waking up. Giving up smoking may improve the quality of your sleep, and it will certainly help the quality of your health.

The bottom line, really, is that if you want to sleep well—and ultimately restore your energy levels—there are a lot of habits you may need to examine and change. The healthier you get, the better you'll sleep.

FOLLOWING THROUGH

- Go to bed only when you feel sleepy; that way, you'll avoid tossing and turning.
- If you find you can't get to sleep, don't fight it. Just get up; go to a different room; and read, watch TV, or listen to music until you feel sleepy.
- Reserve your bedroom for sleep and sex—not for eating, working, or anything else.
- Create a restful, peaceful environment in your bedroom, free of clutter and distractions.
- Keep your bedroom well ventilated and cool. A cool temperature can help you get to sleep and stay asleep.
- Try taking a warm bath an hour or two prior to bedtime. Putting some lavender salts into the bathwater can make the bath more relaxing.
- Experiment with "white noise." Some people need gentle sounds in the background as they drift off to sleep. You might try running a fan or purchasing a sound spa, a device that generates sounds such as a running brook or ocean surf. These are helpful for many people.
- Try some "sleep snacks." Before going to bed, eat something healthy, such as a banana, figs, a bit of turkey, or yogurt. These foods are naturally high in an amino acid called tryptophan, which is helpful for inducing sleep.
- Schedule your workouts early in the day. I typically do my workouts in the morning, and from what I understand about sleep, that's good timing. If you exercise too late in the day—close to bedtime—it will be harder to fall asleep. That's because adrenaline and other hormones are elevated after exercise, and these hormones keep your body revved up—not what you want if you're ready to turn in for the night.
- If you must get up at night, try not to turn on any lights (use a night-light). Exposure to light in the middle of the night can interfere

with your body's production of melatonin, a hormone that regulates sleep/wake cycles.

PUT MORE QUIETNESS INTO YOUR LIFE

When I was a kid in school, the teachers used the phrase, "It needs quietness." Nowadays, I think that phrase seems so fitting to the way we should try to live. Most of us live our lives as if the bottom is falling out. We're stretched for time. We're rushing around. We're overworked and overwrought. I know what I'm talking about; I've lived it. In tennis, those of us who reach the quarters and semis often have barely enough time to practice, rest, travel, eat, sleep, and play. We're so busy that we sometimes forget to slow down and "smell the roses," as the saying goes. In short, we're fatigued and stressed out.

Stress comes in many guises and disguises. It's a tiny word used in almost every field imaginable, from medicine to engineering to business, and let's not forget sports. For my purpose, though, the dictionary definition is perfect: The mental, emotional, or physical strain caused by anxiety, pressure, constant worry, and nervous tension.

Unless you deal with it, the stress of living a hectic life can keep growing and growing, leading to a buildup of stress hormones that begins to interfere with the body's natural healing ability. A good example of what I'm talking about is Liezel Huber, one of the best doubles players on the circuit today. She injured herself shortly after winning the women's doubles at Wimbledon and was recovering when Hurricane Katrina hit.

Liezel and her husband, Tony, who live in Houston, immediately took it upon themselves to lend a helping hand. They adopted more than 10 families and began the task of finding them shelter, food, and clothing. She also launched a campaign to enlist everyone she knew to offer support to these families during their time of need. Such great enthusiasm, dedication, and love for her fellow Americans were remarkable. Even so, her efforts took a toll. Sometimes you can give too much of yourself, and your body pays the price.

A few weeks into her activities, I contacted her to see how she was doing. Although she was in great spirits, her body was giving her warning signs that she was overdoing it. She sounded and felt as if she was getting the flu. Luckily, things later calmed down enough, and enough support came in from others, that she could give herself a little more time for her body to recover from her wonderful display of compassion.

Some of the cumulative effects of ongoing stress are fatigue, sleep problems, and poor health. Over time, a high level of stress can weaken tendons and ligaments, thin bones, cause muscle spasms, elevate blood pressure, increase cholesterol production, and disrupt digestion, among many other negative effects.

Given the damage that stress can do to us, we need to put more quietness into our lives, wouldn't you say?

One of my favorite plays is *The Search for Signs of Intelligent Life in the Universe*, a one-woman show starring Lily Tomlin. Among the many memorable characters she plays is a woman who wanted the job, wanted the husband, wanted the kids, wanted the perfect life. She was so busy that she wanted to attend a seminar on how to better organize your life and make yourself more efficient, but she couldn't find the time to go! At one point in the play, she laments, "Had I known what having it all was going to be like, I might have settled for less!"

I'm sure you can relate; I know I can. Years ago, I didn't pay as much attention to my family as I could have or should have because I was playing, playing, playing. Sometimes before a big match, I'd even discourage friends from dropping in so I could focus and not have my peace of mind interrupted. Or I would have friends come and hang out with me, but I'd pay no attention to them. Tennis can be a very selfish business. You're always worrying about what you need to do for yourself; forget other people. Everyone has to adjust to your schedule. These days, I'm much more balanced. I know I need to work out, but I also want to have fun, so I might cut my workout time down a little or reschedule an appointment. Some things can wait. Most of the constraints we have are self-imposed, anyway.

Like a lot of people, I used to have a lot of stress because I couldn't say no. I wanted to please everybody. Now I'm better at saying no because I know what my limits are. I just say, "No, I'm not able to," and I don't give any long explanations. I'm nice about it, but I can be pretty firm at the same time.

At other times in my life, I've been under strain because I hadn't learned the value of delegating responsibilities. You can't always do it all. There's no shame in asking some-body to help you. My advice? Let them know what's going on in your life so they understand what you're dealing with. Simply say, "I'd like to know if you'd be willing to help me by doing this." We can all put some control back into our lives by learning how to delegate—and life will be far less overwhelming when we do.

So you see, no one is exempt from the tentacles of stress. I'll share with you one more example, something personal that hit me hard. I'm sure you'll be able to relate because it deals with a breakup between two people, a love affair that went down the drain. It was a relationship in which someone used my affections in order to hold onto a certain lifestyle. That cut deep. I can't tell you the amount of stress I experienced during that time. Every day, I woke up wondering how the day would end. The effect it had on my game and my health, along with the emotional roller coaster I was experiencing, was almost suffocating. I couldn't eat, sleep, or even talk at times. I had bad dreams. I was a basket case. To me, it was the hardest and most important lesson in how to deal with stress.

How did I overcome it? Well, to be honest, it wasn't easy, but it actually happened after a very wise woman came to see me and suggested that I turn my self-pity from a negative force into a more positive force. She taught me how to examine a situation and break it down into workable parts or steps so that I didn't feel overwhelmed.

Basically, you make a plan, enlist the right people for support, and then move forward—slowly at first, but forward nevertheless. You get some perspective, too. Sometimes we turn everything into an end-of-the-world scenario, making "a mountain out of a molehill," or we worry about things over which we have no control. It's better to get a realistic grip on the situation and ask yourself, "How much difference will this situation make in my life a year from now? Will I even remember it? What's the worst thing that could happen? How likely is that to occur?" When you dissect a situation and put a more rational spin on it, you minimize the effect stress has on you.

With this in mind, I took control of my behavior and my emotions. Remember this point, because it is extremely, extremely important: You can be in control of only *you*, not others, so don't let, lease, or turn over control to anyone else or think you can control their behavior. As I learned how to break down my stressors, I became more in control of my actions and reactions, and soon the bad dreams disappeared. I also learned a great deal about myself and the tools I needed to enlist in order to deal with future stressors.

Someone who always had great wisdom about how to channel stress was Billie Jean King. She used to say, "Champions adjust to the situation. And they keep playing until they get it right." You could see it in her game, too. Right in the middle of a match, she would totally change it. If she made a mistake or failed to play up to her potential, she'd make the necessary adjustments and move on.

If something isn't going your way, go a different way. You may have to do less and do it well rather than try to do it all and not do anything well. I know it's a cliché, but don't try to fit a square peg into a round hole. Adjust: Either invent a new way to do it or find the round peg!

Let's say you pledged to jog 10 miles a week, but last week you jogged only 3, and you haven't even hit the pavement this week. You may need to adjust by revising your goal downward. Too often, people stop dead in their tracks because they didn't meet the original goals they set for themselves. Don't stress over it. Your best bet is to switch to plan B—a more realistic goal—and do it. For example, if your goal to jog 10 miles a week isn't working, maybe you need to change your goal to 5 miles a week or try a different activity that's easier to accomplish. Goals are not set in stone; they can be changed.

I've often found, too, that very few people are happy or satisfied with where they are in life or what they have. Most are postponing happiness. You've heard people say, "I'll be happy when I get a job . . . when I get out of college . . . when I get married . . . when I have kids . . . when I get promoted."

What about right now?

Once you decide that today, right where you are now, is a good place to be, you'll begin to appreciate and take advantage of everything you have. The future can take care of itself. Whenever I find myself getting stressed out, I stop and thank my lucky stars. I remind myself that I have made a good living, and I'm free, personally and professionally, to do whatever I want. I know I can still work hard, compete, follow my dreams, reach for the best, and make a positive difference in the world—all without becoming stressed out. It's all a matter of balance and perspective. Remember the word *present.* And remember that to be in the present is actually a present in itself. To be alive, to have another day, is an opportunity to do something. It is, in fact, a present.

Though I've let stress get the better of me more often than I care to admit, someone whose memory keeps me going every day is my grandmother, Grandma Subertova. She was the voice of approval that I still hear in the back of my mind, the person who loved me whether or not I had a good day at the tennis courts or finished my homework or cleaned my room. She just loved me and encouraged me to enjoy life. There is so much to be learned from those whose experience is greater than ours. Think about it: If you wanted to learn how to paint, you'd take lessons from an artist. If you wanted to learn how to speak another language, you'd take a class from a foreign language teacher. If you wanted to learn how to play tennis, you'd go to a seasoned tennis coach. Some of the best lessons you can learn about life come from those who have lived long lives, such as your grandparents or the grandparents of friends.

Another grandmother—the grandma of a very close friend—taught me a treasured lesson about life. When Grandma Layton was a little girl, she used to hate to travel because the family had so much luggage to transport on the train. There were so many suitcases that a porter had to lug every one of them. That's how they had to travel in those days.

Later in life, after she grew up, Grandma Layton still traveled, but there was a difference. All she took with her was a small carry-on. On one trip, she ran into a conductor who had known her when she was a little girl traveling with her family. Surprised, he said, "Where's all your luggage? You carry so little!"

"In my travels and in my life," she told him.

You see, she left it all behind—emotional baggage and otherwise. What about you? Have you packed too much emotional luggage? How much do you really need? Is there stuff you can discard, that isn't really necessary? It's up to you what your baggage is; you pack it.

Whenever I feel the walls closing in on me, I know my life's too crowded with unnecessary stuff, whether it's relationship problems, business issues, tennis, family, or politics. I can do only so much, and I can handle only so much. I start paring down what I can. I start unpacking my emotional luggage and traveling light. Suddenly, the stress isn't there anymore—and I begin to feel so much better.

FOLLOWING THROUGH

- Try forms of exercise that offer mental as well as physical benefits, such as yoga or tai chi.
- Take a breather. One of the quickest and easiest ways to relieve stress is to breathe deeply. When you're under stress, your breathing becomes shallow, whereas deep breathing brings about a cascade of positive changes throughout your body. It slows your heart rate, lowers your blood pressure, and eases anxiety. To try deep breathing, breathe in and out slowly. Let your stomach expand as you inhale and deflate as you exhale. Your shoulders should be relaxed and naturally rise and fall with each deep breath.
- Focus your attention. Instead of doing it all— starting a load of laundry, making dinner,

and reading the mail—do one thing at a time. You won't feel so overwhelmed, and you'll do a better job with whatever you're concentrating on. Also important: You don't have to be a superhero every day. Sometimes just getting the kids to soccer practice on time is an accomplishment. Instead of worrying about whatever you don't get done, recognize that you're doing the best you can and pat yourself on the back for your efforts.

- Prioritize. Decide what activities are most important to you by making a list of your priorities. On your list might be spending more time with your partner, getting involved in your kids' activities, volunteering, exercising, taking care of your diet, and

traveling. Then work on those priorities. If you ever find yourself working on something that's not on your list, stop, course-correct, and get back to the priorities. You only waste a lot of precious time, plus increase your stress level, when you're not focused on your priorities.

- Get a pet. One of the best stress relievers doesn't come from the drugstore; it comes from a pet store or an animal shelter. Many, many studies suggest that having a pet significantly lowers heart rate and blood pressure, especially when you're under stress. With 15 dogs and 12 cats, I should be pretty well buffered from stress!

- Talk it out. Tell your close friends and loved

MEDICAL CAUSES OF FATIGUE

In 1982, I had a frightening illness that came at exactly the wrong time—right before the U.S. Open. My glands swelled to about three times their normal size—from my neck to my armpit and into my chest. When I wasn't sleeping, I just wanted to lie down and read a book. I felt exhausted just getting out of a chair. It was as if somebody had turned the hourglass upside down; I could just feel the sand trickling away. During my matches, just chasing balls took so much out of me that I didn't

have enough strength to do anything when I got to them. After many, many medical tests— some of which thankfully ruled out leukemia—I was diagnosed with toxoplasmosis, an infection caused by a parasite that weakens people and is much more common than anybody realizes. The disease is also called cat virus because you can contract it from exposure to cat feces, but you can also get it from eating contaminated or undercooked meat.

Where did I get it? A cat I had come in contact with was tested

and found not guilty, so my doctors blamed it on an undercooked hamburger I had eaten. I bring this story up to make you aware that there are medical causes behind many cases of fatigue. If you are having trouble pinning down and resolving your tiredness, please, by all means, go to your doctor. Fatigue is often a symptom of the following health problems, among others: anemia (lack of iron in the blood), thyroid disease, diabetes, depression, and chronic fatigue syndrome.

ones about the stress you're going through instead of keeping it bottled up. Also, take a hard look at your life expectations to make sure they're realistic. I have also found that by expressing my thoughts to people in my support system, I not only feel more in control but also gain feedback and insight into the situation so that I can resolve it in a positive manner.

- Have fun. We can all tweak our lives in the direction of more fun and less work, but we don't. When I first came to America, one of the first people I met was a Czech guy who left the country in 1948 and became a dentist in Florida. He was pulling in good money, and I asked him why he and his wife never took a vacation. It turned out he was worried about making more money, although he was already very wealthy. I was stunned. You can't take it with you, but we sure act as if we can.

    Life is not all fun and games, of course, but you should have some fun. I think we can all take a tip from dolphins. They spend 75 percent of their time playing and the rest foraging for food, and even the foraging is like a game to them.

    One of the messages I like to send to everyone, young or old, is to enjoy what you're doing, regardless of what it is. Let the kid in you come out. If you're not having fun, go do something else, unless you absolutely have to pay the mortgage or need a few years to make some money. But ultimately, do what you love and love what you do.

- Control the things you can while letting go of the things you cannot. You'll find that your stress levels drop dramatically when you just let go.

- Prepare for the most likely scenario, and then deal with changes as they arise. Focus on the positives, the good things that are happening, without dismissing the negatives (otherwise, they will get stronger and become stumbling blocks). It's like playing a match while keeping track of what's working and what isn't and then responding accordingly. Most of all, believe in yourself. You can do it!

- Finally, just keep your head up and keep taking those baby steps forward. I really like the saying "That which does not kill you makes you stronger." So look at difficult periods and situations as opportunities—yes, opportunities—to challenge yourself. The more you are able to assess the situation, break it down into possibilities, and test a solution or solutions, the easier it will be to overcome other challenges lying in wait. If you take one problem at a time, one solution at a time, one step at a time, you can handle anything.

    I don't have all the answers to conquering fatigue, and there's certainly no sure-cure answer, since we're all different. But if you're tired of being tired, there's probably an imbalance in your life. You have too many things sapping your energy, such as poor nutrition and exercise habits, sleep problems, and unresolved stress, and not enough good things boosting your energy. If you can make some key changes in your diet, exercise habits, sleep patterns, stress, and life outlook, then over time you'll feel your vitality growing. Don't be surprised if your life gets recharged with a new sense of purpose, accomplishment, and meaning.

PART 2

THE SHAPE YOUR SELF NUTRITION AND EXERCISE PLANS

About 10 years ago, I wrote a series of mystery novels featuring a former tennis champion turned amateur detective as the heroine. These days, I am no longer doing mysteries, but I would like to help you solve the mystery of how to get healthier and more fit. With this in mind, here are my easy-to-follow nutrition and exercise plans that put together what I've talked about so far. As every detective knows, persistence pays off. Do your best to stick to these plans, and you will start feeling strong and energetic in no time. Good nutrition and an active lifestyle may not make you look 20-something, but they just may make you feel that young again.

CHAPTER 8

THE SHAPE YOUR SELF NUTRITION PLAN

I've been in the twilight of my career longer
than most people have had careers.

Since I was a kid, I've always enjoyed going to movies of all kinds: foreign films, old films, comedies, dramas, documentaries. I had read about the *Super Size Me* documentary, and I finally got to see it. When I did, it really hit me how much effect food has on our well-being and how much it can harm or heal us.

Maybe you saw this movie, too. It's the personal story of filmmaker Morgan Spurlock and a "nutrition" experiment he conducts on himself. Although trim and fit at 185 pounds, Spurlock decides to chow down on only McDonald's food for 30 days to see what this regimen does to his body. He will have his meals supersized if asked, and, like two-thirds of Americans, he decides not to work out, on the grounds that the average American avoids exercise. Prior to the beginning of the experiment, he goes to a trio of doctors for a full checkup, and they pronounce him in excellent health.

After a week, Spurlock has gained about 10 pounds. He gets depressed. By the end of the 30 days, he has gained about 25 pounds. His cholesterol is sky-high. He has headaches and nausea. His sex life is nonexistent, and his liver is close to failing. Not surprisingly, his doctors are shocked by his declining health after only 1 month of eating this food.

After watching this movie—which I think should be recommended viewing before you take another bite of your favorite fast food!—I got a real sense of why obesity has become one of our nation's biggest health problems. We've gotten so far away from healthy eating, preferring junk food and fast food instead, that we're getting very fat and very sick in the process.

Thus, in this chapter, I will give you some great ideas for delicious meals, snacks, and all kinds of other yummy stuff that is actually good for you. So many times, when I am eating my "grub," people with me are curious about it. When I tell them what it is, they ooh and ahh or say, "That sounds too healthy for me." Then I give them a taste, and they exclaim, "Wow, this is delicious!"

The meal plans and recipes that follow will give you a great start toward improving the quality of your life. After all, we have only one trip around in life that we know of for sure, and we should make the most of it. One place to start is with what you put on your plate.

EATING TO SHAPE YOUR SELF

No single food provides all the nutrients your body needs for good health. That's why eating a variety of wholesome foods from different food groups helps ensure that you get the necessary nutrients to help you get fit and hopefully stay that way. I'm basing my guidelines on the way I eat and on what is now being widely recommended nutritionally to get you to your ideal weight, provide energy, delay aging, and promote resistance to some diseases. What follows are the nutritional building blocks of a healthy diet that will help you reach these goals.

Vegetables: 2 or 3 Servings (or More) Daily

Veggies have loads of nutrients, including vitamin C, beta-carotene, riboflavin, iron, calcium, fiber, and more. I don't mean to get too technical and boring by talking about nutrients, but I just want to remind you that vegetables are good for you, so bear with me. And, if you don't drown them in cream sauces, margarine, or dips, vegetables are low in fat and calories. I don't think you can eat too many vegetables, but if you're not a vegetable lover, start gradually at the lower range of 2 servings a day or try at least one fresh vegetable juice a day.

One way to guarantee variety and high nutrition is to buy vegetables in lots of different colors, as well as to juice combinations of vegetables. Here are some examples.

Dark green, leafy vegetables. The greener the leaf, the more anti-aging compounds it contains. That's why I think it's smart eating to enjoy one mixed salad a day. I love greens and eat a lot of them. A few years back, I ordered a salad that supposedly contained 14 different types of greens. Curiosity got the best of me, so I counted the leaves in the salad, and I think I found 12 kinds. You certainly don't have to make salads with that much variety, but do try to include more of the following in your diet.

Arugula

Beet greens

Bok choy

Broccoli

Chicory

Collards

Dandelion greens

Endive

Kale

Lettuce (all varieties)

Mustard greens

Parsley

Spinach

Swiss chard

Turnip greens

Watercress

Yellow, red, and orange vegetables. Colorful veggies are proven fighters of aging, cancer, and heart disease because they contain a boatload of nutrients, including antioxidants. Try to include several servings of the following in your diet each week.

Carrots

Pumpkin

Tomatoes

Winter squash

Yellow and red bell peppers

Starchy vegetables. I'm sold on these because they keep my energy "batteries" charged up. Higher in healthy carbs, they contain more natural goodness than most processed carbs.

Corn

Potatoes

Sweet potatoes

Yams

Other vegetables. Veggies are probably the best fuel you can put in your body, when you get right down to it. I'm always trying new vegetables, so I never get bored with my diet. Here's a list of some of my favorites.

Alfalfa sprouts

Artichokes

Asparagus

Avocado*

Brussels sprouts

Cabbage (all varieties)

Cauliflower

Celery

Cucumber

Eggplant

Garlic

Hearts of palm

Kohlrabi

Leeks

Mushrooms

Okra

Onions

Pea pods

Peppers (all varieties)

Radishes

Scallions

Snow peas

Sprouts

String beans

Summer squash (all varieties)

Yellow beans

Zucchini

Avocado is technically considered a fruit. Sometimes called a superfood, it's an excellent source of nutrients, including healthy fats, that you might not get elsewhere. I use avocados in many of my recipes.

Fruits: 2 or 3 Servings Daily

Like veggies, fruits contain plenty of nutrients to keep your body on the beam. The more fruits you include in your diet, the less likely you are to develop practically every major disease. How about that? The same cannot be said for Twinkies!

Each day, try to include at least 1 serving of fruit that is high in vitamin C. Round out your choices with other selections. If fruit smoothies appeal to you as they do to me, try whirring several of your favorite fruits in a blender with a little juice, fat-free or soy yogurt, and maybe some ice. Smoothies are fun and flavorful, not to mention loaded with nutrition.

Fruits High in Vitamin C

Black currants

Citrus fruits (oranges, grapefruit, tangerines, and tangelos)

Kiwifruit

Melons

Strawberries

Fruits High in Beta-Carotene

Apricots

Cantaloupe

Mangoes

Nectarines

Papayas

Peaches

Other Nutritious Fruits

Apples

Bananas

Blackberries

Blueberries

Boysenberries

Cherries

Cranberries

Figs (fresh or dried)

Grapes

Guavas

Pears

Persimmons

Pineapple

Plantains

Plums

Pomegranates

Prunes

Raspberries

Power Carbs: 2 or 3 Servings Daily

I realize that carbs have a less-than-sterling reputation these days. Yet the carbs I list below are healthy, highly nutritious foods or, as some call them, good carbs. I prefer to call them power carbs because they energize the body for exercise and daily life, plus supply lots of B vitamins, minerals, and plenty of fiber for good digestive health. I have grouped these carbs into breads, cereals, grains, and pastas. In each grouping, you'll find the best ones to put in your body.

Breads

Low-fat whole wheat pancakes

Whole grain, pumpernickel, or rye bread

Whole grain bagels

Whole grain dinner rolls

Whole grain hamburger or hotdog buns

Whole wheat crackers

Whole wheat English muffins

Whole wheat flour tortillas or corn tortillas

Whole wheat pitas

Cereals

Cooked buckwheat groats

Cooked corn grits

Cooked Farina, Cream of Wheat, or other
hot cereal

Low-fat granola

Minimally processed high-fiber cereal,
such as Fiber One, All Bran, or Kashi
Go Lean

Muesli

Cooked oat bran

Cooked oatmeal

Wheat germ

Grains

Basmati rice

Bulgur wheat

Couscous

Long-grain brown rice

Millet

Pearled barley

Quinoa

Wild rice

Pasta

Egg noodles

Soba noodles

Somen (Japanese) noodles

Spinach or other vegetable pasta

Whole wheat pasta

**Dairy Foods and Substitutes:
2 or 3 Servings Daily**

We've all been told that these foods are great
sources of calcium and other nutrients. But
they also taste great when blended with super-
nutritious fruit for a low-cal, healthy snack,
dessert, or quick meal. If you take some frozen
fruit, for example, and whir it in the blender
with milk, nut milk, or yogurt, it turns into a
big, creamy milkshake that comes in at around
150 to 200 calories. Compare that with a real
shake—a medium one—which has more than
400 calories but doesn't contain other good
stuff, like fiber.

If you're like me, and your body doesn't get
along with dairy products, choose alternatives
such as nut milks and grain milks. To me, these
taste better than regular dairy milks anyway,
and you can buy them in enriched versions to
pump up your nutrition. Here's a list of dairy
foods and dairy substitutes from which to
choose.

Almond or other nut milk

Enriched plain soy milk

Fat-free or low-fat Lactaid milk

Fat-free or 1% milk

Hard cheese

Low-fat, sugar-free yogurt

Low-fat acidophilus milk

Low-fat or fat-free cheese

Plain yogurt

Reduced-fat cottage cheese

Rice milk

Soy yogurt

Low-Fat Proteins:
2 or 3 Servings Daily

Athletes like to talk a lot about protein: how much you need for good performance, muscle conditioning, staying power, and so forth. But I think sometimes they overestimate its value. Protein is important, but it isn't as huge a staple as most athletes make it out to be. I've found that protein should merely complement what is the real nutritional force in any meal: plant-based foods like fresh vegetables, whole grains, and fruit. Even so, you definitely need a reasonable serving of protein at each of your main meals. It helps the fuel you get from carbs last longer. When I eat the right balance of protein and carbs, I feel like I can stay on the court forever.

You can get healthy protein from both vegetarian sources and low-fat animal sources. Vegetarian proteins like beans, lentils, and soy foods (tofu and tempeh, for example) are a whole lot better for you than many meats because they supply a nearly complete set of disease-preventing nutrients, without all the fat. But if you can't stomach vegetarian proteins all

the time, choose low-fat animal proteins such as fish and white-meat poultry over high-fat cuts of meat. Dairy foods and dairy substitutes supply protein, too. It just makes good sense to cut down on fatty meats and stick with high-fiber, low-fat foods if you want to stay well as you get older.

Vegetarian Proteins: Beans and Legumes

Black beans

Black-eyed peas

Broad beans (fava beans)

Chickpeas (garbanzo beans)

Cranberry beans

Great Northern beans

Kidney beans

Lentils

Lima beans

Navy beans

Pink beans

Pinto beans

Split peas

White beans

Other Vegetarian Proteins

Eggs

Egg whites

Tempeh

Tofu

Vegetarian burgers/patties

Bass

Catfish

Clams

Cod

Crab

Flounder

Grouper

Haddock

Halibut

Lobster

Mahi mahi

Monkfish

Orange roughy

Oysters

Perch

Red snapper

Salmon

Shrimp

Sole

Tilapia

Trout

Tuna

Whitefish

When I have the option at a seafood store or restaurant, I get wild salmon instead of farm-raised salmon. The farm-raised type is a little iffy because it is supposedly contaminated with more toxins and chemicals than wild salmon caught in the northern Pacific Ocean.

There are also unsafe levels of mercury in some fish, including swordfish, king mackerel, and certain kinds of tuna (one of the most popular fish we eat). Mercury levels in tuna can vary: Fresh tuna steaks and canned white albacore tuna, for example, have higher levels than canned light tuna. Although fish and shellfish can be an important part of a healthy diet, keep your intake to about 12 ounces a week of a variety of types that are lower in mercury. These include shrimp, canned light tuna, salmon, and catfish.

Animal Proteins: Poultry

Ground chicken breast

Ground turkey breast

Low-fat turkey bacon

Low-fat turkey sausage

Skinless chicken breast

Skinless Cornish hen

Skinless turkey breast

Healthy Fats: 1 Serving Daily

Fats always seem to get a bad rap, but I have learned that there are actually healthy fats you can include in your diet. Basically, healthy choices are unsaturated, which is nutritional lingo that describes the chemical makeup of the fat. Really, all you need to know is that there's plenty of proof showing that these fats, which are listed below, are good for you in the right amounts.

Canola oil

Flaxseed oil

Light or soy mayonnaise

Low-fat salad dressings

Macadamia nut oil

Nut butters

Nuts and seeds, such as almonds, Brazil nuts, pecans, walnuts, pumpkin seeds, sesame seeds, and sunflower seeds

Olive oil

Peanut oil

Sesame oil

Walnut oil

PICTURE YOUR SERVING SIZES USING EVERYDAY OBJECTS

I remember the first time I came to the States in 1973, and I went into a 7-Eleven store to buy some food. Back then, sodas were sold in 6-ounce portions. Guess what the average portion size is today? Twenty ounces! I sampled my first hamburger then, too. That's when burgers were about $2\frac{1}{2}$ ounces; today, they're double, even triple, that size! It's no wonder people are becoming so overweight these days.

Okay, how do you know a reasonable serving of food when you see it? Try to visualize the everyday objects listed in "Easy Ways to Figure Your Serving Sizes" on page 116 when planning your meals, eating out, or grabbing a snack. For example, the amount of meat I recommend as part of a healthy meal is about 4 ounces, and that's about the same size as your

checkbook or an audiocassette tape. This system will help you control your portions so you don't eat too much or too little.

THE SHAPE YOUR SELF NUTRITIONAL GUIDELINES

- The following sample meal plans are meant to be used as a guide and starting point for planning your own meals, not as a strict regimen. My intent is to provide an example of a healthy diet that is also delicious. When foods taste great, as these do, you're more likely to enjoy them and keep eating this way. Feel free to substitute foods you like or leave out what you don't like. If you're a vegetarian, choose vegetarian proteins over animal proteins. This plan is very flexible.
- The serving size guidelines are easy to remember and make meal planning a breeze: Each day, you'll choose 2 or 3 servings from each food group, with the exception of fats (1 serving daily). Check "Easy Ways to Figure Your Serving Sizes" on page 116 to see what constitutes a serving.
- If you're trying to lose weight or control your weight, choose the lower number of servings each day—2 servings of a particular food rather than three, for example.
- If you're not accustomed to having a lot of veggies, fruits, or juices, gradually introduce them into your meals.
- Use fresh fruits and vegetables whenever you can.
- Enjoy fruit for dessert or as a snack. Veggies make great snacks, too.

- Choose whole grain breads, cereals, and pastas.
- Try to have at least one fresh juice daily. Gradually add more juices and/or smoothies into the plan as snacks or with meals. Fresh juice gives you an instant energy boost, and you won't crash from it as you would after eating a candy bar or doughnut. Whenever I want to feel good, I have a juice. To me, it's a legal high.
- Eat breakfast every day. Skipping breakfast may make your metabolism sluggish, heighten hunger later in the day, and possibly lead to weight gain.
- If you limit your intake of dairy products, as I do, use nuts and nut milks. Both are high in bone-saving calcium. Or take advantage of calcium-fortified soy and grain milks.
- Use condiments in moderation, both with meals and in recipes. Condiment serving sizes are generally no more than 2 tablespoons. It's fine to use sweet condiments such as honey or maple syrup, but again, use small amounts, no more than a tablespoon or two a day.
- Keep yourself well hydrated by drinking water throughout the day, especially on active days. I like putting stuff in my water to spice it up, such as good old lemons, sliced cucumber, mint, or whatever suits my taste buds.
- Savor your food by eating slowly. This gives your stomach a better chance to register that it is full, so you won't overeat and may stop before you actually clean your plate.

THE SHAPE YOUR SELF BREAKFAST OPTIONS

Always enjoy a glass of fresh juice to start your day, or 1 serving of any fresh fruit. Then choose one of the following breakfasts.

Breakfast #1: Vegetable and Cheese Omelet (see recipe on page 118) or 3 scrambled egg whites with a dairy serving

1 slice whole grain bread

Breakfast #2: 1 serving organic cereal of choice with 1 cup fat-free or 1% milk, soy milk, grain milk, Almond Milk (see recipe on page 118), or yogurt

Breakfast #3: 2 whole wheat pancakes with 1 tablespoon maple syrup

2 strips vegetarian or turkey bacon

1 cup fat-free or 1% milk, soy milk, grain milk, Almond Milk, or yogurt

Breakfast #4: 1 slice whole grain toast topped with 1 ounce cheese and 1 tomato slice (broil until cheese begins to melt)

Breakfast #5: 1 tablespoon nut butter and jelly on whole grain toast

Breakfast #6: Egg white and bacon sandwich (2 scrambled egg whites and 2 slices turkey or soy bacon placed in a whole wheat English muffin or whole grain bagel to form a sandwich)

Breakfast #7: 1 serving any hot cereal (oatmeal is my favorite) with 1 tablespoon chopped nuts and 1 cup fat-free or 1% milk, soy milk, grain milk, Almond Milk, or yogurt

EASY WAYS TO FIGURE YOUR SERVING SIZES

STANDARD SERVING SIZES	EVERYDAY OBJECT EQUIVALENTS
VEGETABLES (2 OR 3 SERVINGS DAILY)	
2 cups mixed greens	is 2 baseballs
1 cup raw vegetables	is a baseball
½ cup cooked vegetables	is a cupcake or muffin wrapper full
1 medium baked potato or sweet potato	is a computer mouse
8 to 10 oz vegetable juice	is a ¾-full to almost-full soda can
FRUITS (2 OR 3 SERVINGS DAILY)	
1 medium piece of raw fruit	is a tennis ball
1 cup berries or chopped fruit	is a baseball
¼ cup dried fruit	is a golf ball
8 to 10 oz fruit juice	is a ¾-full to almost-full soda can
POWER CARBS (2 OR 3 SERVINGS DAILY)	
Breads	
A serving of whole grain, pumpernickel, or rye bread	is 1 slice
½ whole grain 3 oz bagel	is a hockey puck
½ whole wheat English muffin	is a hockey puck
½ whole grain hamburger bun	is a hockey puck
1 whole wheat pita	is an average-size saucer
1 medium whole grain dinner roll	is a tennis ball
4 whole grain crackers	are 4 tea bags
1 whole wheat flour tortilla or corn tortilla	is an average-size saucer
2 low-fat whole wheat pancakes	are 2 compact discs (CDs)
Cereals	
½ cup cooked cereal	is a cupcake or muffin wrapper full
½ cup muesli or low-fat granola	is a cupcake or muffin wrapper full
1 cup minimally processed high-fiber cereal	is a baseball
4 Tbsp wheat germ	is 4 checkers

STANDARD SERVING SIZES	EVERYDAY OBJECT EQUIVALENTS
Grains	
½ cup cooked rice	is a cupcake or muffin wrapper full
½ cup cooked bulgur wheat	is a cupcake or muffin wrapper full
½ cup cooked couscous	is a cupcake or muffin wrapper full
DAIRY FOODS AND SUBSTITUTES (2 OR 3 SERVINGS DAILY)	
1 cup milk (fat-free, 1%, Lactaid, acidophilus, soy, rice, and nut milks)	is a baseball
1 cup plain, low-fat, or sugar-free yogurt or soy yogurt	is a baseball
½ cup reduced-fat cottage cheese	is a cupcake or muffin wrapper full
1 oz hard cheese	is a lipstick tube
2 oz low-fat or fat-free cheese	is 2 lipstick tubes
LOW-FAT PROTEINS (2 OR 3 SERVINGS DAILY)	
Vegetarian Proteins	
½ cup cooked beans/legumes	is a cupcake or muffin wrapper full
½ cup cooked or raw lentils	is a cupcake or muffin wrapper full
1 vegetarian burger/patty	is a mayonnaise jar lid
½ cup tofu	is a cupcake or muffin wrapper full
Animal Proteins	
4 oz fish, chicken breast, turkey breast, or Cornish hen	is a checkbook or audiocassette tape
HEALTHY FATS (1 SERVING DAILY)	
1 tablespoon oil (olive, canola, flaxseed, peanut, sesame, and walnut oil)	is a checker
2 tablespoons low-fat salad dressing or light or soy mayonnaise	is a Ping-Pong ball or 2 checkers
2 tablespoons nuts or seeds	is a Ping-Pong ball or 2 checkers
1 tablespoon nut or seed butters	is a checker

MEAL PLAN *Day 1*

BREAKFAST

Choose from breakfasts listed on page 115.

SNACK

CARROT JUICE or fresh vegetable juice of choice

LUNCH

1 cup organic black bean soup

4 whole wheat crackers

2 cups mixed salad greens with 4 cherry tomatoes and 1 tablespoon low-fat or fat-free dressing

1 cup strawberries with 1 cup low-fat or fat-free plain or sugar-free yogurt

DINNER

4 ounces grilled chicken breast

1 cup steamed spinach or spinach lightly sautéed in 1 teaspoon olive oil

1 medium baked sweet potato

1 serving fruit of choice

VEGETABLE AND CHEESE OMELET

1   teaspoon olive oil

½   cup sliced mushrooms

½   small tomato, chopped

½   small onion, chopped

3   egg whites

2   ounces shredded low-fat cheese

Heat the oil in a nonstick skillet over medium heat. Add the mushrooms, tomato, and onion and sauté for 4 to 5 minutes. Add the egg whites and spread evenly over the vegetables. Cook until the egg mixture is set but the top is still moist. Add the cheese and fold over.

Makes 1 serving

ALMOND MILK

1½   cups raw almonds

4   cups water

Soak the almonds in the water overnight. Process in a blender and strain to remove the almond granules. The result is a delicious, creamy, nutritious milk that can be used on cereal and in smoothies. It can be refrigerated for 3 to 4 days.

Makes about 4 cups

CARROT JUICE

4–5   carrots, washed

Juice the carrots and enjoy!

Makes 1 serving

MEAL PLAN *Day 2*

BREAKFAST

Choose from breakfasts listed on page 115.

SNACK

SOY FRUIT SMOOTHIE

LUNCH

Large tossed tuna salad: 2 cups shredded butter crunch lettuce, ½ cup shredded raw carrots, ½ cup chopped pepper (any kind you like), 3 ounces water-packed tuna, and 1 tablespoon low-fat or fat-free dressing

1 medium orange

DINNER

1 serving PASTA PRIMAVERA (see recipe on page 139)

1 serving fruit of choice

SOY FRUIT SMOOTHIE

- 1   cup plain organic soy milk
- ½   apple, chopped
- ½   cup fresh blueberries
- ¾   cup red seedless grapes
- 1   tablespoon chopped dates

Process the ingredients in a blender until smooth.

Makes 1 large serving

MEAL PLAN *Day 3*

BREAKFAST

Choose from breakfasts listed on page 115.

SNACK

MARTINA'S 8

LUNCH

1 serving **GUACAMOLE WRAPS**

1 to 2 cups raw baby carrots

DINNER

4 ounces grilled or baked salmon

1 cup steamed broccoli

½ to 1 cup brown rice

1 serving **HONEY-BAKED PEARS**

MARTINA'S 8

- 1 tomato
- 1 carrot
- 1 stalk celery
- 1 cup or handful spinach
- ½ cucumber
- 1 red bell pepper
- 1 cup broccoli
- 1 cup cabbage
- 1 slice fresh ginger

Juice the ingredients and enjoy.

Makes 1 serving

GUACAMOLE WRAPS

- 1 large avocado
- 1 small tomato, chopped
- 1 jalapeño pepper, finely chopped
- 2 tablespoons chopped onion
- 2 tablespoons fresh cilantro, finely chopped
- 4 ounces Cheddar cheese, shredded
  Salt and black pepper to taste
  Tabasco or other hot sauce, optional (I like a little extra kick)
- 1 head butter crunch lettuce

Slice the avocado lengthwise and remove the pit. (I do this by sticking the blade of the knife into the pit and twisting.) Scoop the pulp into a medium bowl and mash thoroughly with a fork. Add the tomato, jalapeño, onion, cilantro, cheese, salt, pepper, and hot sauce, if desired. Mix well. Mound the mixture in lettuce leaves and roll into burrito-style wraps.

Makes 2 servings

HONEY-BAKED PEARS

- 4 medium pears
- 2 tablespoons raisins
- 2 tablespoons nuts, chopped
- $\frac{1}{3}$ cup honey
- 1 teaspoon ground cinnamon

Preheat the oven to 350°F. Coat a shallow baking dish with cooking spray. Peel the pears, cut in half, and core. Arrange cut side up in baking dish. In a small bowl, mix together the raisins and nuts. Fill the pears with the mixture, pour on the honey, and sprinkle with cinnamon. Bake for about 25 minutes, or until tender.

Makes 4 servings

MEAL PLAN *Day 4*

BREAKFAST

Choose from breakfasts listed on page 115.

SNACK

BANANA SOY SMOOTHIE

LUNCH

CAESAR TOFU SALAD

1 whole grain dinner roll

1 serving fruit of choice

DINNER

1 cup organic vegetarian chili

1 cup mixed salad greens with 4 cherry tomatoes and 1 tablespoon low-fat or fat-free dressing

BANANA SOY SMOOTHIE

- 1 cup plain organic soy milk
- 1 banana, peeled and frozen
- 1 tablespoon honey
- 1 tablespoon peanut butter, optional (I love to spice this smoothie up with it)

Process the ingredients in a blender until smooth.

Makes 1 serving

CAESAR TOFU SALAD

- 2 cups romaine lettuce, washed and torn
- ½ cup cubed tofu
- ¼ cup chopped red onion
- 2 anchovy fillets, optional
- 2 black olives, pitted and chopped
  Salt and black pepper to taste
- 2 tablespoons light Caesar dressing

Place the lettuce on a plate and top with the tofu, onion, anchovies (if desired), olives, salt, and pepper. Drizzle with the dressing.

Makes 1 serving

MEAL PLAN *Day 5*

BREAKFAST
Choose from breakfasts listed on page 115.

SNACK
CARROT-BEET JUICE or other fresh vegetable juice of choice

LUNCH
Veggie or garden burger on whole grain hamburger bun with 1 teaspoon mustard, ketchup, or both

1 cup mixed salad greens with sliced red bell pepper and 1 tablespoon low-fat or fat-free dressing

1 cup soy milk

1 serving fruit of choice

DINNER
4 ounces baked turkey breast

1 medium baked potato

1 cup steamed summer squash

1 serving fruit of choice

CARROT-BEET JUICE

2 carrots, washed
1 beet, with greens
½ cucumber

Juice the ingredients and enjoy.

Makes 1 serving

MEAL PLAN 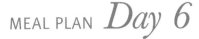 *Day 6*

BREAKFAST

Choose from breakfasts listed
on page 115.

SNACK

APPLE-VEGGIE JUICE
or other fresh vegetable
juice of choice

LUNCH

1 serving MARTINA'S RED
LENTIL SALAD

1 serving fruit of choice

1 cup low-fat or fat-free plain
or sugar-free yogurt

DINNER

Vegetarian chef's salad:
4 ounces soy ham (diced) and
2 ounces soy cheese (diced),
served over a bed of mixed
salad greens and assorted
salad vegetables with 2 tablespoons low-fat dressing

1 serving fruit of choice

APPLE-VEGGIE JUICE

2 apples, cored
4 medium carrots, washed
½ lemon
1 slice fresh ginger

Juice the ingredients and enjoy.

Makes 1 serving

MARTINA'S RED LENTIL SALAD

1 cup dried red lentils
½ cup pearled barley
½ cup dried chickpeas
1 cup grape tomatoes
1 cup pea pods, chopped
3 tablespoons fresh cilantro, or to taste
3 tablespoons olive oil
Salt and black pepper to taste

Place the lentils, barley, and chickpeas in a large bowl with enough
water to cover generously and soak overnight. Drain and transfer to
a large salad bowl. Add the tomatoes, pea pods, and cilantro. Add
the oil, salt, and pepper and toss. (You can add other raw vegetables
as desired. I like sun-dried tomatoes, corn, avocado, and baby corn.)

Makes 4 servings

MEAL PLAN *Day 7*

BREAKFAST

Choose from breakfasts listed on page 115.

SNACK

1 to 2 cups chopped raw vegetables dipped in **HERBED YOGURT CHEESE**

LUNCH

1 cup organic vegetable soup

4 whole wheat crackers

1 serving fruit of choice

DINNER

1 serving **VEGETABLE STIR-FRY** (see recipe on page 143)

½ to 1 cup brown rice

1 cup strawberries with 1 cup low-fat or fat-free plain or sugar-free yogurt

HERBED YOGURT CHEESE

4 cups plain yogurt
Fresh chopped herbs, such as garlic, basil, oregano, and rosemary, to taste

Line a strainer with a coffee filter and spoon in the yogurt. Place the strainer over a bowl, cover with plastic wrap, and refrigerate overnight. The whey will drain out of the yogurt and leave creamy yogurt cheese, which can be used on baked potatoes, as a spread on toast or crackers, or as a dip for raw vegetables. Add a few pinches of herbs.

Makes about 1 cup

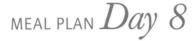

BREAKFAST

Choose from breakfasts listed on page 115.

SNACK

RASPBERRY–ALMOND MILK SMOOTHIE

LUNCH

Greek salad: 1 cup mixed baby greens, 3 sliced black olives, 2 tablespoons chopped onion, 4 slices tomato, 2 ounces feta cheese, 1 tablespoon olive oil, and 2 to 3 tablespoons balsamic vinegar

1 whole grain dinner roll

1 serving fruit of choice

DINNER

1 serving **PASTA GENOVESE WITH PESTO SAUCE**

1 cup mixed salad greens with 4 cherry tomatoes and 1 tablespoon low-fat or fat-free dressing

RASPBERRY–ALMOND MILK SMOOTHIE

- 1 cup Almond Milk (see recipe on page 118)
- 1 cup fresh or frozen organic raspberries
- 1 teaspoon honey, optional

Process the ingredients in a blender until smooth. (Frozen berries are often cheaper and are as nutritious as fresh.)

Makes 1 serving

PASTA GENOVESE WITH PESTO SAUCE

- ½ cup olive oil
- ½ cup fresh basil, chopped
- 1 clove garlic, minced, optional
- 1 teaspoon salt
- ¼ teaspoon black pepper
- ¼ cup pine nuts (lightly toasted, if desired)
- ¼ cup Parmesan cheese
- 3 cups cooked hot or cold whole wheat pasta

In a blender, process the oil, basil, and garlic (if desired), on high. Let stand for 15 minutes.

Add the salt, pepper, and pine nuts and blend at a lower setting. Add the cheese and blend. Serve over pasta. (This sauce keeps in the refrigerator for a week and can be frozen. It makes a great standby dish. If you're desperate for a lower-calorie version, you can replace the oil with water or vegetable or chicken broth and the pine nuts with walnuts. I've often done this. To thicken the sauce, add some parsley along with the basil.)

Makes 6 servings

MEAL PLAN *Day 9*

BREAKFAST

Choose from breakfasts listed on page 115.

SNACK

MANGO SMOOTHIE (see recipe on page 136)

LUNCH

EASY ITALIAN SUB (see recipe on page 140)

1 cup low-fat or fat-free plain or sugar-free yogurt

DINNER

CHICKEN KEBAB

CHICKEN KEBAB

½ cup pineapple juice
3 tablespoons teriyaki sauce
1 tablespoon olive oil
2 cherry tomatoes
1 boneless, skinless chicken breast, cut into large chunks
2–3 chunks fresh pineapple
2–3 chunks green or red bell pepper

In a shallow dish, combine the pineapple juice, teriyaki sauce, and oil. Alternate the tomatoes and chicken, pineapple, and pepper chunks on a skewer. Dip in the marinade, coating well, and discard the marinade. Cover and refrigerate the kebab for 30 minutes. Grill or broil until the chicken is cooked through and the vegetables and fruit are cooked. Remove from the skewer and serve. (You may double or triple this recipe for additional servings.)

Makes 1 serving

BREAKFAST

Choose from breakfasts listed on page 115.

SNACK

SALAD IN A GLASS or other fresh vegetable juice of choice

LUNCH

Hummus pita: 4 tablespoons hummus, ½ cup shredded lettuce, 4 slices cucumber, and 2 slices tomato in 1 whole wheat pita

1 serving fruit of choice

1 serving **SMOOTHIE POP**

DINNER

4 ounces baked whitefish (any type)

1 cup cooked carrots

1 cup baby spinach with 1 ounce feta cheese (crumbled), 1 tablespoon raisins, 1 tablespoon sliced almonds, and 1 tablespoon low-fat or fat-free raspberry vinaigrette dressing

1 serving fruit of choice

SALAD IN A GLASS

- 2 carrots, washed
- 3 stalks celery
- 5 romaine lettuce leaves
- ½ cucumber

Juice the ingredients and enjoy.

Makes 1 serving

SMOOTHIE POPS

- 1 cup low-fat yogurt
- 1½ teaspoons vanilla extract
- 1 teaspoon lemon juice
- ¼ cup honey
- 1 cup chopped fresh fruit, such as blueberries, raspberries, and cantaloupe

Process the ingredients in a blender until smooth. Pour into four ½-cup ice-pop molds and insert wooden sticks. Cap the molds and freeze for at least 4 hours.

Makes 4 servings

MEAL PLAN *Day 11*

BREAKFAST

Choose from breakfasts listed on page 115.

SNACK

BANANA ROLL

LUNCH

Vegetarian BLT: 2 slices vegetarian bacon, 2 slices tomato, lettuce, and 1 teaspoon soy or light mayonnaise on 2 slices whole wheat bread

1 serving fruit of choice

DINNER

1 serving **TOFU ROLL-UPS**

Fresh Herb Salad: ¼ package mixed salad greens; ½ cup fresh basil leaves, chopped; ¼ cup fresh parsley, chopped; assorted chopped salad vegetables; and 1 tablespoon low-fat or fat-free vinaigrette

BANANA ROLL

- 2 teaspoons honey
- 2 tablespoons Nutella
- 1 medium banana
  Ground cinnamon
- 2 tablespoons wheat germ, toasted

Spread the honey and Nutella on the banana and sprinkle lightly with cinnamon. Roll the banana in the wheat germ until coated. Refrigerate or eat right away.

Makes 1 serving

TOFU ROLL-UPS

- 1 pound soft tofu
- 2 egg whites
- ¼ cup plus 3 tablespoons fat-free Parmesan cheese
- 1 cup fancy shredded fat-free mozzarella cheese
- 1 tablespoon sweet basil
- 2 teaspoons dried oregano
- 1 teaspoon garlic salt
- ¼ teaspoon red pepper
- ¼ teaspoon black pepper
- 10 cooked whole wheat lasagna noodles
- 1 can (26¾ ounces) light spaghetti sauce

Preheat the oven to 350°F.

In a medium bowl, blend the tofu, egg whites, ¼ cup Parmesan, mozzarella, basil, oregano, garlic salt, red pepper, and black pepper until the mixture resembles a paste. Lay a lasagna noodle on a piece of foil and spread 3 tablespoons of the tofu mixture up to the edge. Repeat with the other noodles, then roll up and cut each roll in half.

Fill a large rectangular baking dish with the spaghetti sauce. Add the rolls and sprinkle with the remaining Parmesan. Cover and bake for 45 minutes.

Makes 5 servings

MEAL PLAN *Day 12*

BREAKFAST

Choose from breakfasts listed on page 115.

SNACK

ENERGY BALLS (I usually eat 2, which is enough to get me going)

LUNCH

MEDITERRANEAN SALAD (see recipe on page 145)

1 whole grain dinner roll

1 serving fruit of choice

DINNER

4 ounces grilled chicken

1 cup steamed vegetable of choice

½ cup cooked corn

ENERGY BALLS

⅓ cup honey

¼ cup plain organic soy milk

1 cup old-fashioned oatmeal

1 tablespoon sesame seeds

¼ cup nuts, finely chopped

4 dried figs, chopped (you may need to soak these in water until they are pliable)

Coconut flakes

In a saucepan over high heat, combine the honey and soy milk. Bring to a boil and cook for 1 minute. Set aside.

In a blender, food processor, or juicer, process the oatmeal, sesame seeds, nuts, and figs until finely ground. Add to the honey mixture. Form into balls and dust with the coconut flakes.

Makes 14 to 16 balls

MEAL PLAN *Day 13*

BREAKFAST

Choose from breakfasts listed on page 115.

SNACK

RASPBERRY–ALMOND MILK SMOOTHIE (see recipe on page 126)

LUNCH

Tuna sandwich: 3 ounces tuna mixed with 1 tablespoon soy mayonnaise on 2 slices dark rye bread

Assorted raw vegetables

1 serving fruit of choice

DINNER

1 serving SALSA SALAD

1 serving PEACH TART

SALSA SALAD

- 2 cups corn
- 1½ cups drained cooked kidney beans or 1 can (15 ounces) kidney beans, rinsed and drained
- 1 large tomato, finely chopped
- 1 green bell pepper, finely chopped
- 1 small onion, finely chopped
- 1 tablespoon fresh cilantro, finely chopped
- 1 clove garlic, minced
- 2 tablespoons white balsamic vinegar
- 1 tablespoon olive oil
  Salt and black pepper to taste

In a large bowl, mix the ingredients. Refrigerate until chilled.

Makes 4 servings

PEACH TART

- 2 cups pecans, finely minced
- 1 cup dates, finely minced
- ½ teaspoon vanilla extract
- 1 teaspoon cinnamon
- 4–5 ripe peaches, peeled, pitted, and sliced into thin wedges
- 1 tablespoon fresh lemon juice
- ⅓ cup honey
  Ground cinnamon to taste

In a food processor or blender, process the pecans, dates, vanilla, and cinnamon. Spread and press the mixture into the bottom and up the sides of a 9-inch tart pan to form the crust. Arrange the peach slices over the crust and drizzle with the lemon juice. Drizzle the honey over the peaches and sprinkle with cinnamon. Serve immediately.

Makes 6 to 8 servings

MEAL PLAN *Day 14*

BREAKFAST

Choose from breakfasts listed on page 115.

SNACK

CUCUMBER COCKTAIL or other fresh vegetable juice of choice

LUNCH

1 cup organic black bean soup

4 whole wheat crackers

2 cups mixed salad greens with 4 cherry tomatoes and 1 tablespoon low-fat or fat-free dressing

1 cup strawberries with 1 cup low-fat or fat-free plain yogurt

DINNER

4 ounces grilled chicken breast

1 cup steamed spinach

1 medium baked sweet potato

1 serving fruit of choice

CUCUMBER COCKTAIL

1 cucumber, cut into chunks

3 apples, cored

Juice the ingredients and enjoy.

Makes 1 serving

MEAL PLAN *Day 15*

BREAKFAST

Choose from breakfasts listed on page 115.

SNACK

1 serving fruit of choice

LUNCH

Greek salad: 1 cup mixed baby greens, 3 sliced black olives, 2 tablespoons chopped onion, 4 slices tomato, 2 ounces feta cheese, 1 tablespoon olive oil, and 2 to 3 tablespoons balsamic vinegar

1 whole grain dinner roll

1 serving fruit of choice

DINNER

1 serving BEAN FAJITAS

BEAN FAJITAS

1 cup drained cooked black beans
2 whole wheat flour tortillas
½ cup chopped fresh zucchini
1 small onion, chopped
1 tomato, chopped
2 tablespoons low-fat shredded cheese
2 tablespoons low-fat or fat-free sour cream, optional

Heat the beans. Mound on the tortillas and top with the zucchini, onion, tomato, cheese, and sour cream (if desired). Roll up burrito style.

Makes 2 servings

BREAKFAST

Choose from breakfasts listed on page 115.

SNACK

SPICY JUICE or other fresh juice of choice

LUNCH

CAESAR TOFU SALAD

(see recipe on page 122)

DINNER

4 ounces grilled or baked salmon

1 cup steamed broccoli or other vegetable

½ to 1 cup brown rice

1 serving fruit of choice

SPICY JUICE

2   pears, cored
1   apple, cored
2   oranges
¼   teaspoon ground cinnamon

Juice the pears, apple, and oranges. Pour into a tall glass and sprinkle with the cinnamon.

Makes 1 serving

MEAL PLAN *Day 17*

BREAKFAST
Choose from breakfasts listed on page 115.

SNACK
CABBAGE COOLER or other fresh juice of choice

LUNCH
MEDITERRANEAN SALAD (see recipe on page 145)

1 whole grain dinner roll

1 serving fruit of choice

DINNER
4 ounces baked turkey breast

1 medium baked potato

1 cup steamed summer squash

1 serving **BERRY PARFAIT**

CABBAGE COOLER

4 carrots, washed
6 leaves cabbage
1 slice fresh ginger

Juice the ingredients and enjoy.

Makes 1 serving

BERRY PARFAIT

1½ cups fresh raspberries or blueberries
3 tablespoons honey
2 cups plain yogurt
1 teaspoon vanilla extract

In a blender, process the berries and 1 tablespoon honey until smooth. Strain through a fine sieve. In a small bowl, combine the yogurt with the vanilla and remaining honey. Layer the yogurt and berry puree in 4 parfait glasses.

Makes 4 servings

BREAKFAST

Choose from breakfasts listed on page 115.

SNACK

MANGO SMOOTHIE

LUNCH

1 serving **MARTINA'S RED LENTIL SALAD** (see recipe on page 124)

1 serving fruit of choice

DINNER

4 ounces grilled tuna

1 cup steamed green beans with 1 tablespoon slivered almonds

½ to 1 cup mashed butternut squash

MANGO SMOOTHIE

1 cup finely chopped fresh mango

¼ cup orange juice

1 cup crushed ice

Process the ingredients in a blender and enjoy.

Makes 1 serving

MEAL PLAN *Day 19*

BREAKFAST

Choose from breakfasts listed
on page 115.

SNACK

MOCK WINE or other fresh
juice of choice

LUNCH

Tuna sandwich: 3 ounces
tuna mixed with 1 tablespoon
soy or light mayonnaise on
2 slices dark rye bread

Assorted raw vegetables

1 serving fruit of choice

DINNER

Organic vegetarian chili

1 cup mixed salad greens
with 4 cherry tomatoes and
1 tablespoon low-fat or fat-
free dressing

1 serving fruit of choice

MOCK WINE

2 cups sweet seedless grapes
1 cup blueberries
2 stalks celery

Juice the ingredients and enjoy.

Makes 1 serving

BREAKFAST

Choose from breakfasts listed on page 115.

SNACK

1 serving GINGERY JUICE or other fresh juice of choice

LUNCH

Turkey sandwich: 3 ounces baked turkey or 2 fat-free turkey slices, 1 slice Swiss cheese, lettuce, and 1 teaspoon Dijon mustard on 2 slices whole grain bread

Assorted raw vegetables

1 serving fruit of choice

DINNER

1 serving MAPLE-GLAZED SALMON

1 cup steamed asparagus

1 sliced fresh tomato

GINGERY JUICE

4–5 carrots
1 large apple, cored
1 slice fresh ginger (1 inch thick)
Juice of 1 lemon

Juice the carrots, apple, and ginger and stir in the lemon juice.

Makes 2 servings

MAPLE-GLAZED SALMON

3 tablespoons pure maple syrup
2 tablespoons teriyaki sauce
½ teaspoon cornstarch
4 pieces salmon fillet (about 5 ounces each)

Preheat the oven to 475°F. Lightly coat a shallow baking dish with cooking spray.

In a small bowl, whisk the syrup, teriyaki sauce, cornstarch, and 1 tablespoon cold water. Place the salmon skin side down in the baking dish and drizzle with the glaze. Bake, basting once with the glaze, for about 15 minutes, or until the fish flakes easily when tested with a fork.

Makes 4 servings

MEAL PLAN *Day 21*

BREAKFAST

Choose from breakfasts listed on page 115.

SNACK

8 to 10 ounces fresh vegetable juice of choice

LUNCH

Crab-stuffed pita: 3 ounces canned crabmeat, 1 tablespoon low-fat mayonnaise, 1 chopped celery stalk, and 2 slices tomato in a whole wheat pita

1 serving fruit of choice

DINNER

1 serving PASTA PRIMAVERA

1 serving fruit of choice

PASTA PRIMAVERA

1 tablespoon olive oil
2 cloves garlic, minced
1 cup chopped carrots
1 cup coarsely chopped broccoli florets
1 cup finely chopped zucchini
1 jar artichoke hearts, chopped
1 cup chopped mushrooms
1 red bell pepper, chopped
1 cup chopped onion
⅓ cup dry white wine
2 tablespoons minced fresh basil
2 tablespoons minced fresh oregano
½ teaspoon salt
¼ teaspoon black pepper
12 ounces whole wheat pasta
½ cup grated Asiago or fresh Parmesan cheese

Heat the oil in a large nonstick skillet over medium-high heat. Add the garlic and carrots and sauté for 5 minutes. Add the broccoli, zucchini, artichokes, mushrooms, bell pepper, onion, wine, basil, oregano, salt, and pepper and cook just until tender.

Meanwhile, cook the pasta according to package directions. Drain well and set aside.

Spoon about 1 cup of the vegetables over each serving of pasta and top with 1 tablespoon of cheese.

Makes 6 to 8 servings

BREAKFAST

Choose from breakfasts listed on page 115.

SNACK

8 to 10 ounces fresh vegetable/fruit juice of choice

LUNCH

EASY ITALIAN SUB

1 cup low-fat or fat-free plain or sugar-free yogurt

DINNER

4 ounces grilled chicken breast

1 cup steamed spinach

1 medium baked sweet potato

1 serving fruit of choice

EASY ITALIAN SUB

- 2   tablespoons Pesto Sauce (see recipe on page 126)
- 1   whole grain hot dog roll or small submarine roll
- 1   Roma tomato, sliced
- 2   slices part-skim mozzarella cheese

Spread the pesto sauce on both sides of the roll and add the tomato and cheese.

Makes 1 serving

BREAKFAST

Choose from breakfasts listed on page 115.

SNACK

BANANA SOY SMOOTHIE (see recipe on page 122)

LUNCH

Vegetarian BLT: 2 slices vegetarian bacon, 2 slices tomato, lettuce, and 1 teaspoon soy or light mayonnaise on 2 slices whole wheat bread

1 serving fruit of choice

DINNER

1 serving **EGGPLANT PARMESAN**

1 cup mixed salad greens with 4 cherry tomatoes and 1 tablespoon low-fat or fat-free dressing

EGGPLANT PARMESAN

- ½ cup low-fat or fat-free Parmesan cheese
- 1 eggplant, peeled, sliced into ¼-inch pieces, and patted dry
- 1 clove garlic, minced
- 1 teaspoon Italian seasoning
- 1 jar light spaghetti sauce or tomato puree

Preheat the oven to 400°F. Coat a nonstick baking pan with cooking spray.

Place the cheese in a shallow dish and dip the eggplant slices to coat. Coat both sides of the slices with cooking spray. Place on the baking pan and sprinkle with the garlic and Italian seasoning. Bake for 6 to 8 minutes.

Transfer to a baking dish. Spread the spaghetti sauce over the eggplant and return to the oven for about 5 minutes, or until heated through.

Makes 4 servings

BREAKFAST

Choose from breakfasts listed on page 115.

SNACK

1 cup chopped fresh fruit tossed with 1 cup low-fat or fat-free plain or sugar-free yogurt

LUNCH

1 serving PORTOBELLO MUSHROOM SANDWICH

1 serving fruit of choice

DINNER

4 ounces baked whitefish (any type)

1 cup cooked carrots

1 cup baby spinach with 1 ounce feta cheese (crumbled), 1 tablespoon raisins, 1 tablespoon sliced almonds, and 1 tablespoon low-fat or fat-free dressing

PORTOBELLO MUSHROOM SANDWICHES

1 teaspoon olive oil
2 tablespoons balsamic vinegar
4 tablespoons fresh basil, finely chopped
2 portobello mushrooms
2 whole grain buns
2 slices part-skim mozzarella cheese
Sliced onions, optional
Sliced tomatoes, optional

In a small bowl, combine the oil, vinegar, and basil. Brush the mushrooms with the oil mixture, place on a broiler pan, and broil for 5 minutes on each side, or until tender. Lightly toast the buns. Place the mushrooms and cheese in the buns and add the onions and tomatoes, if desired.

Makes 2 servings

MEAL PLAN *Day 25*

BREAKFAST

Choose from breakfasts listed on page 115.

SNACK

1 serving TROPICAL PUDDING

LUNCH

Greek salad: 1 cup mixed baby greens, 3 sliced black olives, 2 tablespoons chopped onion, 4 slices tomato, 2 ounces feta cheese, 1 tablespoon olive oil, and 2 to 3 tablespoons balsamic vinegar

1 whole grain dinner roll

DINNER

1 serving VEGETABLE STIR-FRY

½ to 1 cup brown rice

TROPICAL PUDDING

1 cup mango chunks
1 banana
1 teaspoon tahini (sesame paste)

Process the ingredients in a blender until smooth.

Makes 2 servings

VEGETABLE STIR-FRY

¾ teaspoon cornstarch
2 tablespoons soy sauce
½ teaspoon sugar
1 tablespoon sesame or peanut oil
1 clove garlic, minced
2 slices fresh ginger, minced
2 cups broccoli florets
½ cup sliced celery
1 can bamboo shoots
1 cup bean sprouts
1 small onion, cut into thin wedges
　Hot sauce, red curry powder, or other hot spice, optional

In a small bowl, combine the cornstarch and 2 tablespoons cold water. Stir in the soy sauce and sugar and set aside.

Heat a large skillet or wok over high heat and add the oil. Add the garlic and ginger and sauté for 1 minute. Add the broccoli, celery, bamboo shoots, sprouts, onion, and hot sauce, if desired. Stir-fry for about 5 minutes, or until vegetables are crisp-tender. Stir in the reserved soy sauce mixture and cook, stirring, for 1 minute, or until the vegetables are well coated. (The vegetables listed above are my suggestions, but any vegetables can be used in a stir-fry. Experiment!)

Makes 4 servings

BREAKFAST

Choose from breakfasts listed on page 115.

SNACK

RASPBERRY–ALMOND MILK SMOOTHIE (see recipe on page 126)

LUNCH

Hummus pita: 4 tablespoons hummus, ½ cup shredded lettuce, 4 slices cucumber, and 2 slices tomato in 1 whole wheat pita

1 serving fruit of choice

DINNER

1 serving VEGETABLE FRITTATA

1 serving POTATO PANCAKES

VEGETABLE FRITTATA

2	tablespoons olive oil
2–3	cups chopped yellow bell peppers, onions, mushrooms, broccoli, and zucchini
1	tablespoon fresh basil, chopped
6	eggs
2	tablespoons fat-free milk
½	cup grated Parmesan cheese
	Salt and black pepper to taste

Preheat the oven to 350°F. In a 9- or 10-inch ovenproof skillet, warm the oil. Add the vegetables and basil and sauté just until soft.

In a small bowl, combine the eggs and milk. Pour over the vegetables and sprinkle with the cheese, salt, and black pepper. Cook over medium heat for 2 to 3 minutes, or until the eggs are set. Bake until the top of the frittata is no longer runny.

Makes 2 to 3 servings

POTATO PANCAKES

4	cups grated potatoes
1	cup grated onion
1	egg or two egg whites
¼	cup parsley, finely chopped
	Herbed Yogurt Cheese (see recipe on page 125) or low-fat or fat-free sour cream

Preheat the oven to 375°F. Coat a baking sheet with cooking spray.

In a medium bowl, combine the potatoes, onion, egg or egg whites, and parsley. Spoon about 2 tablespoons onto the baking sheet and flatten to form a pancake. Repeat with the remaining mixture. Bake for about 20 minutes on each side, or until crisp. Top with the yogurt cheese or sour cream.

Makes 4 servings

MEAL PLAN *Day 27*

BREAKFAST

Choose from breakfasts listed on page 115.

SNACK

8 to 10 ounces fresh vegetable juice of choice

LUNCH

MEDITERRANEAN SALAD

1 serving fruit of choice

DINNER

1 cup organic vegetarian chili

1 cup mixed salad greens with 4 cherry tomatoes and 1 tablespoon low-fat or fat-free dressing

1 serving fruit of choice

MEDITERRANEAN SALAD

    2 cups romaine lettuce, torn or shredded
    ½ cup chickpeas
    2 ounces feta cheese
    ½ cup chopped cucumber
    ½ small onion, chopped
    2 black olives
    2 tablespoons chopped fresh basil
    1 tablespoon olive oil
    2 teaspoons balsamic vinegar

In a salad bowl, make a bed of lettuce and arrange the chickpeas, cheese, cucumber, onion, olives, and basil on top. Toss with oil and vinegar.

Makes 1 serving

MEAL PLAN *Day 28*

BREAKFAST

Choose from breakfasts listed on page 115.

SNACK

8 to 10 ounces fresh vegetable juice of choice

LUNCH

Vegetarian BLT: 2 slices vegetarian bacon, 2 slices tomato, lettuce, and 1 teaspoon soy or light mayonnaise on 2 slices whole wheat bread

1 serving fruit of choice

DINNER

4 ounces grilled or baked salmon

1 cup steamed broccoli or other vegetable

1 serving fruit of choice

Moving plant-based foods to the center of your plate is one of the easiest things you can do to preserve your health—as long as you make it a lifetime commitment. Something I've found helpful is making creativity and experimentation with new foods and recipes an ongoing habit in my life. Most of us can live longer and better by eating for our personal best. I'm willing to practice what I preach. Are you? I hope so!

Bon appétit!

CHAPTER 9

THE SHAPE YOUR SELF
EXERCISE PLAN

Had I not been a tennis pro, I would have been an athlete of some other kind, because I like to move; I like to test the limits of my body while it's still capable of pushing the limits.

Whether you want to use exercise to help you lose weight, perform better, get more active than you are now, or just feel better, period, this plan is going to help you do it. What I love about these workouts is that they are fun—not to mention convenient. With a few inexpensive exercise toys, you can turn a small part of your home or workspace into a gym and work out according to your schedule.

You can incorporate some tweaks and variations into many of these exercises that will make them more challenging. Instead of just increasing the number of repetitions and sets, you can change an exercise slightly to make it harder as you get stronger. This progressive quality—with increases in levels of difficulty and challenge—makes the exercises more interesting. They are never, ever boring. If they were, I wouldn't be doing them, and they wouldn't be in this book.

The principle behind the exercises and workout plan is to stimulate your muscles more than they're accustomed to. Using weights, exercise toys, your body weight, gravity, repetitions, and sequence, you'll gradually increase your fitness level by making each exercise and each workout harder and more challenging.

The exercise toys you will need include:

- A pair of dumbbells (in different weights)
- Exercise tubing (with door attachment)
- Foam roller
- Medicine ball
- Stability ball
- An Xerdisc

These can be purchased at any good sports equipment store and from many Internet sites, such as www.spriproducts.com. However, if you decide not to use exercise toys, you can substitute everyday objects and still get a decent workout. The chart below lists substitutions.

In the exercise descriptions, I often mention "neutral spine" or "neutral alignment." These terms mean essentially the same thing and are popping up everywhere in gyms and exercise classes these days. All they mean is a position (sitting, standing, or moving) in which your spine is not overly arched or rounded but is in its natural S-shaped position. In addition, your body, from head to toe, is aligned as if a plumb line were running from your ears down through your torso and into your legs and feet. Neutral alignment feels natural and requires minimal energy and less muscle activity to maintain.

As you progress, get stronger, feel better, and all that, you will want to keep doing these workouts. Because they are fun, not very demanding time-wise, and simple to follow, it will be easier for you to stick with the program and keep pushing yourself. Of course, when you not only feel the results but see them, you'll be inspired to keep going.

Here is how I would go about getting started. First, check the section on finding your level on page 208. If you are a beginner, read through the exercises first. Study the photos (trainer Lisa Austin and I enjoyed posing for them!). Let the information soak in. This will familiarize you with the moves and how they benefit your body. The more you understand about how the exercises work, the more sense they will make to you. If you are intermediate or advanced, you can pretty much do the exercises right away.

I've given you 4 weeks of workouts for each level. As you finish each one, you will advance to the next level. Take your time; don't push yourself too much. Remember, less is more, especially when you're just getting started. Get a feel for it all, see how your body feels the next day, and then progress to the next level when you're ready.

Okay, have at it—and good luck!

EXERCISE TOY SUBSTITUTES

IF YOU DON'T HAVE THIS:	USE THIS:
Dumbbells	Heavy objects such as books or milk jugs filled with water
Exercise tubing	Dumbbells, surgical tubing, or heavy objects such as books or milk jugs filled with water
Foam roller	Swimming pool noodle
Medicine ball	A properly inflated basketball, soccer ball, or even a football
Stability ball	A firm pillow or a bench, couch, or chair, depending on the exercise
Xerdisc	A couch cushion (to mimic an unstable surface)

CORE EXERCISES

These exercises are designed to strengthen the muscles that support your spine from your lower back to your upper back, your hips to your shoulders. They target the abdominal, hip, and back muscles.

BUN BURNER

START: Lie on your back on an exercise mat or other soft surface, with your feet on the floor, your knees bent, and your arms at your sides.

FINISH: Press both feet into the floor and lift your pelvis. Squeeze your buttocks together, keeping your navel drawn in and your tailbone pulled in slightly to maintain neutral alignment. Hold for 3 to 5 seconds. Breathe naturally as you lower your pelvis back to the floor. On the descent, let your spine slowly touch the mat one vertebra at a time until your tailbone reaches the floor. Perform the recommended number of repetitions.

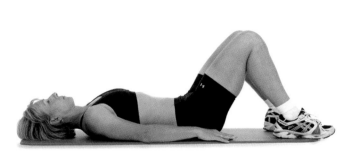

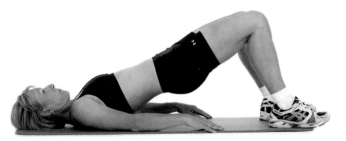

BUN BURNER WITH XERDISC

START: Lie on your back on an exercise mat or other soft surface, with your feet on an Xerdisc, your knees bent, and your arms at your sides.

FINISH: Press both feet into the Xerdisc and lift your pelvis. Squeeze your buttocks together, keeping your navel drawn in and your tailbone pulled in slightly to maintain neutral alignment. Hold for 3 to 5 seconds. Breathe naturally as you lower your pelvis back to the floor. On the descent, let your spine slowly touch the mat one vertebra at a time until your tailbone reaches the floor. Perform the recommended number of repetitions.

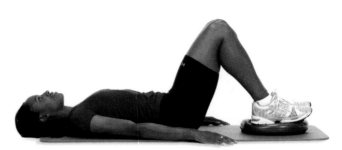

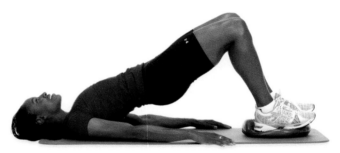

TORSO TONER

START: Kneel and place your hands on the floor, with your shoulders over your wrists and your pelvis over your knees. Maintain neutral alignment, with your shoulders back and your navel pulled in. Lift your right arm and extend it forward.

FINISH: With your right arm still outstretched, extend your left leg out behind you. Then do the exercise with the opposite arm and leg. Continue alternating arms and legs for the recommended number of repetitions. Be careful not to let your pelvis rock out of neutral while lifting your legs.

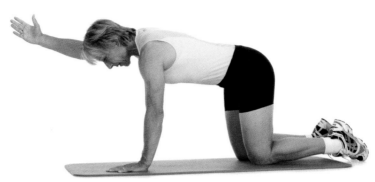

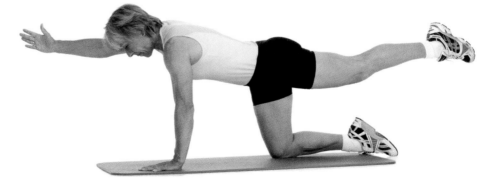

BUN BURNER WITH LEG LIFT

START: Lie on your back on an exercise mat or other soft surface, with your feet on the floor, your knees bent, and your arms at your sides. Lift one foot off the floor and raise your leg with the knee bent at a 90-degree angle.

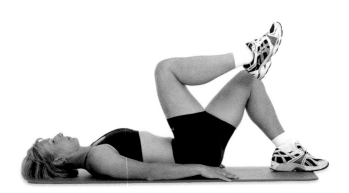

FINISH: Press your other foot into the floor and lift your pelvis. Squeeze your buttocks together, keeping your navel drawn in and your tailbone pulled in slightly to maintain neutral alignment. Hold for 3 to 5 seconds. Breathe naturally as you lower your pelvis back to the floor. On the descent, let your spine slowly touch the mat one vertebra at a time until your tailbone reaches the floor. Perform the recommended number of repetitions, then repeat with the other leg.

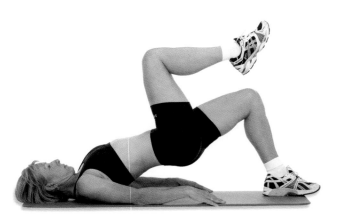

BUN BURNER WITH LEG LIFT ON XERDISC

START: Lie on your back on an exercise mat or other soft surface, with your feet on an Xerdisc, your knees bent, and your arms at your sides. Lift one foot off the Xerdisc and raise your leg with the knee bent at a 90-degree angle.

FINISH: Press your other foot into the Xerdisc and lift your pelvis. Squeeze your buttocks together, keeping your navel drawn in and your tailbone pulled in slightly to maintain neutral alignment. Hold for 3 to 5 seconds. Breathe naturally as you lower your pelvis back to the floor. On the descent, let your spine slowly touch the mat one vertebra at a time until your tailbone reaches the floor. Perform the recommended number of repetitions, then repeat with the other leg.

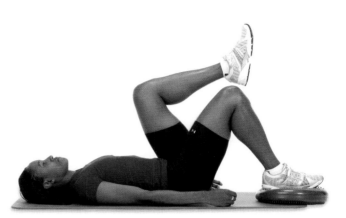

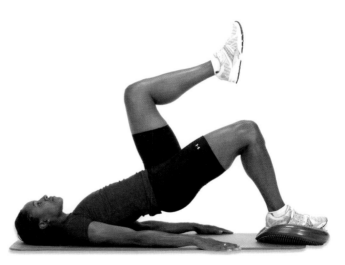

TUMMY TUCK

START: Lie on your back on an exercise mat or other soft surface, with your knees bent and your arms at your sides. Place a tennis ball or Hacky Sack on your navel (optional).

FINISH: Inhale. Then, on the exhale, draw your abdomen in, without performing a crunch, to engage your outer and inner abs. (Using a tennis ball helps you see the drawing-in movement.) Repeat this breathing and movement pattern, using deep, controlled breaths, for the recommended number of repetitions.

TIP: To make this exercise more challenging, perform it with both feet off the floor and your legs raised at 90-degree angles ("dead bug" position). Slowly extend one foot forward to intensify the exercise. Keep your abdomen drawn in and maintain neutral alignment in your pelvis.

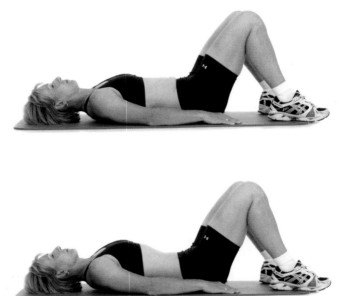

TUMMY TUCK WITH STABILITY BALL

START: Sit on a stability ball with your back straight. Inhale.

FINISH: Then, on the exhale, draw your abdomen in to stimulate your inner abs. Repeat this breathing and movement pattern, using deep, controlled breaths, for the recommended number of repetitions.

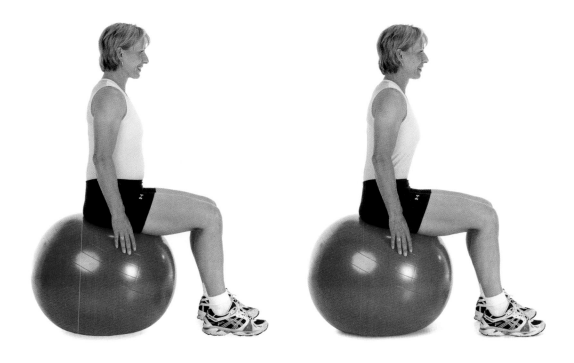

TUMMY TIGHTENER WITH FOAM ROLLER

START: Lie on your back with a foam roller positioned vertically under you and your torso in neutral alignment. Place both feet on the floor with your knees bent, your legs slightly less than hip width apart, and your arms crossed over your chest.

FINISH: With your left foot on the floor, raise your right leg, keeping your knee bent at 90 degrees. Hold for 3 to 5 seconds, then lower your foot to the starting position. Perform the recommended number of repetitions, then repeat with the other leg.

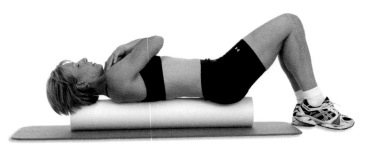

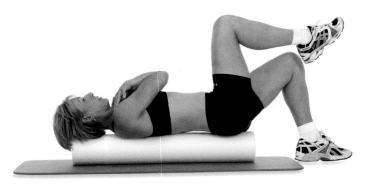

WAIST WHITTLER

START: Kneel on an exercise mat or other soft surface. Lean forward and place your forearms slightly more than shoulder width apart on the mat. Clasp your hands together. Bend your knees and cross your feet at the ankles. Draw in your navel and maintain a neutral spine.

FINISH: Uncross your feet. Place your toes on the floor. Push back, elevating your lower body and torso so that you're in a plank position. Balance with only your forearms and toes. Hold for 30 seconds to 1 minute, then release. Perform the recommended number of repetitions.

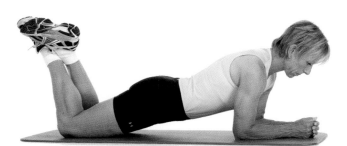

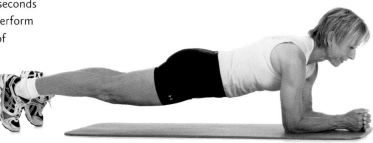

TIP: To make the exercise more challenging, lift one foot off the floor while maintaining the same body position. Balancing your feet or forearms on an unstable surface such as an Xerdisc intensifies this exercise as well.

"DEAD BUG" HEEL TAP WITH FOAM ROLLER

START: Lie on your back with a foam roller positioned vertically under you. Lift both feet off the floor so your legs are raised at 90-degree angles. Keep your arms alongside the roller, your shoulders down, and your navel drawn firmly in.

FINISH: Inhale as you tap one foot on the floor while maintaining a neutral spine. Exhale, then bring your foot back to the starting position. Repeat, alternating legs.

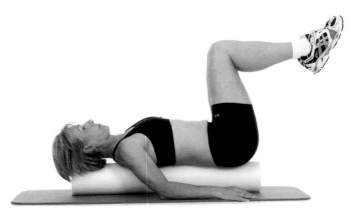

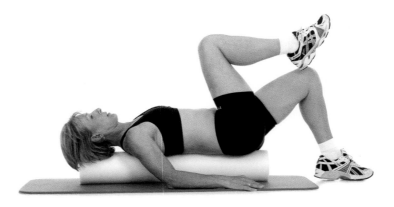

CORE CRUNCHER WITH STABILITY BALL

START: Facing the floor, go into prone position, with your hands about shoulder width apart on the floor and your lower legs on a stability ball. Keep your navel pulled in and your spine neutral. Your inner thighs should be lifted and your legs straight. Draw your shoulders down and squeeze your shoulder blades together. Hold for 30 seconds to 1 minute.

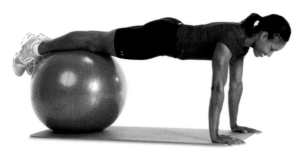

FINISH: Roll the ball underneath you, bringing your knees to your chest and pulling your abs up strongly. Keep your head aligned with your spine and your shoulders down. Walk forward slowly on your hands back to the starting position. (The farther you walk, the greater the intensity of the exercise.) Perform the recommended number of repetitions.

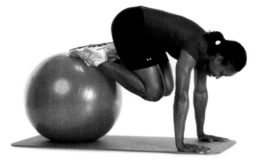

TIP: To make this exercise more challenging, as you bring your knees toward your chest, twist your lower body slightly to one side. Then walk forward slowly on your hands back to the starting position. Repeat on the other side.

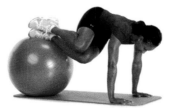

TWIST

START: Attach exercise tubing securely to a post at chest level. Stand and hold the handles on the left side of your body, keeping some tension in the tubing.

FINISH: Inhale and rotate your upper body to the left. On the exhale, rotate to the right without moving your lower body. Keep both hands on the handles, in line with your shoulders. Slowly return to the starting position. Perform the recommended number of repetitions.

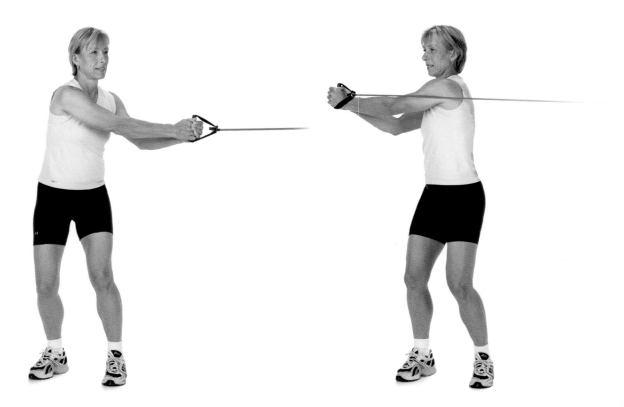

TWIST UP

START: Attach exercise tubing securely to a post at knee level. Stand and hold the handles on the left side of your body, keeping some tension in the tubing.

FINISH: Inhale and rotate your upper body upward and to the right. On the exhale, rotate down to the left without moving your lower body. Slowly return to the starting position. Perform the recommended number of repetitions.

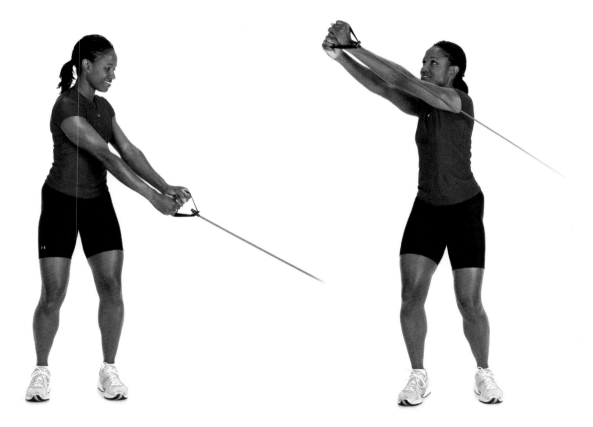

These exercises are considered strength moves because they make you stronger, so you'll be able to bend down and pick things up off the floor without pulling a muscle, have more muscle endurance (staying power) for the sport of your choice, and enhance the shape of your body.

The exercises are meant to be performed on a "progressive continuum," meaning that each exercise is harder than the previous one. Once an exercise feels too easy, after you've done it for a while, it's time to try its more challenging variation.

Lower-Body Exercises

Target muscles: Upper legs (quadriceps, hamstrings), hips, and gluteals

WALL SQUAT WITH STABILITY BALL

START: Place a stability ball in the small of your back, cross your arms over your chest, and lean against a wall.

FINISH: Bend your knees, lowering your hips until your thighs are almost parallel to the floor. Slowly return to the starting position. Perform the recommended number of repetitions.

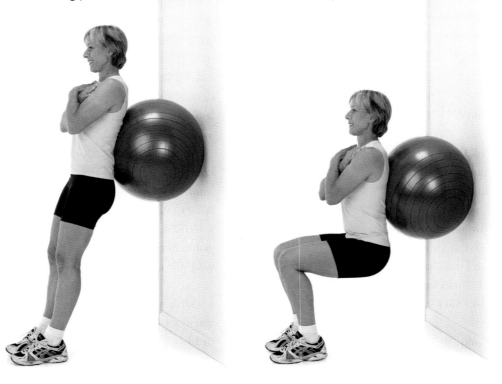

SINGLE-LEG SQUAT

START: To find your balance, stand on one leg (this is your support leg).

FINISH: Keeping your torso upright, bend the knee of your support leg to a 45-degree angle. Be careful to maintain the alignment of your hip, knee, and ankle. Return to the starting position. Perform the recommended number of repetitions.

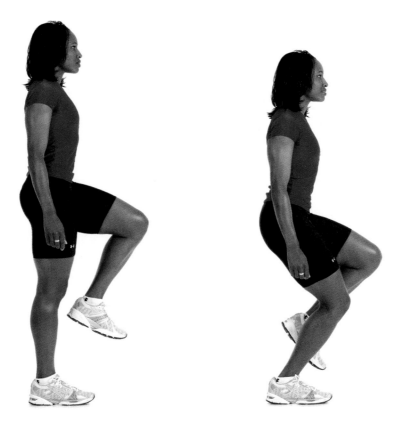

SINGLE-LEG SQUAT WITH XERDISC

START: Stand on an Xerdisc and raise one leg.

FINISH: Keeping your torso upright, bend the knee of your support leg at a 45-degree angle. Be careful to maintain the alignment of your hip, knee, and ankle. Return to the starting position. Perform the recommended number of repetitions.

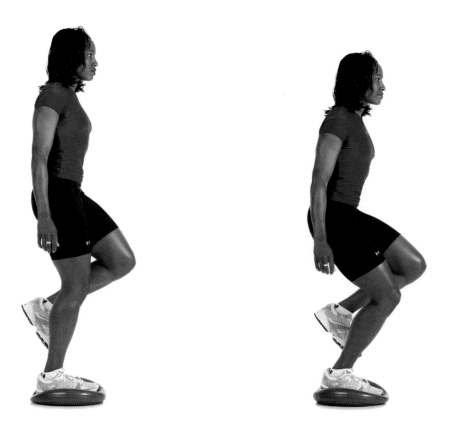

TIP: To make this exercise a bit easier, keep both feet on the Xerdisc and bend your knees to a 45-degree angle.

SPLIT-STANCE SQUAT WITH STABILITY BALL

START: Stand with your right foot forward and your left foot back in a split stance. Place a stability ball in the small of your back and lean against a wall.

FINISH: Keeping your torso upright and your hips in neutral, bend your knees and lower your hips so your thighs are almost parallel to the floor. Pause, then press through both feet back to the starting position. Perform the recommended number of repetitions.

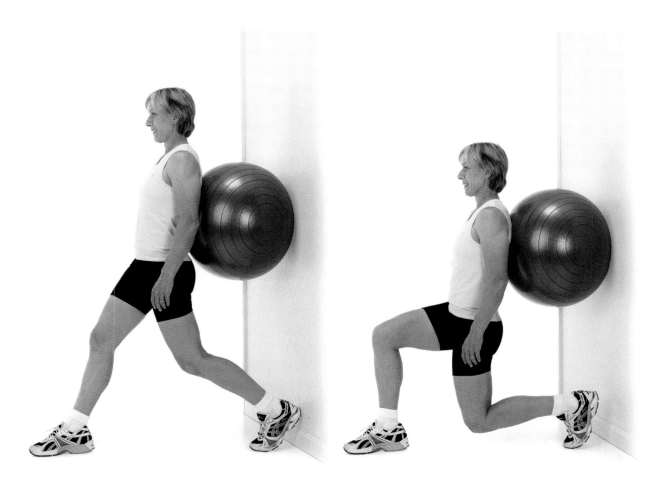

Upper-Body Exercises

Target muscles: Chest (pectorals), backs of upper arms (triceps), and biceps

BENT-KNEE PUSHUP

START: Kneel on an exercise mat or other soft surface. Lean forward and place your hands slightly more than shoulder width apart on the mat. Bend your knees, cross your feet at the ankles, and straighten your arms.

FINISH: Draw in your navel and maintain a neutral spine. Slowly bend your arms and lower your torso toward the floor, keeping your elbows close to your rib cage. Press back up to the starting position. Perform the recommended number of repetitions.

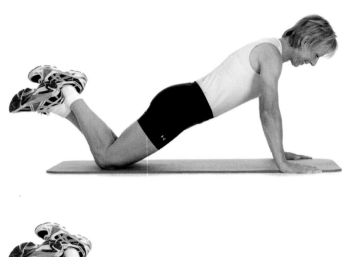

BENT-KNEE PUSHUP ON UNSTABLE SURFACE

START: Kneel on an exercise mat or other soft surface. Lean forward and place your hands slightly more than shoulder width apart on an unstable surface such as Xerdiscs, medicine balls, or a balance board. Bend your knees, cross your feet at the ankles, and straighten your arms.

FINISH: Draw in your navel and maintain a neutral spine. Slowly bend your arms and lower your torso toward the floor, keeping your elbows close to your rib cage. Press back up to the starting position. Perform the recommended number of repetitions.

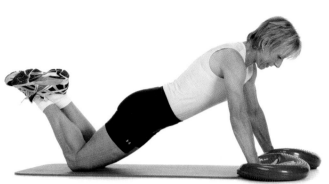

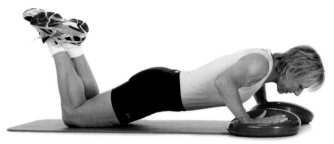

PUSHUP

START: Kneel on an exercise mat or other soft surface. Extend your arms and place your hands slightly more than shoulder width apart on the mat, keeping your arms straight but not locked and your wrists in line with your shoulders. One at a time, extend your legs behind you until you are balanced on the fronts of your feet, with your legs straight and ankles close together. Your body should form a straight line from your head to your heels.

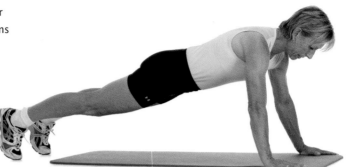

FINISH: Bend your elbows and lower your torso until it is a couple of inches from the floor, with your elbows aligned with your shoulders and your wrists aligned under your elbows. Keep your navel drawn in and maintain a neutral spine. Press back up to the starting position. Perform the recommended number of repetitions.

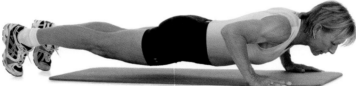

PUSHUP WITH MEDICINE BALLS

START: Kneel on an exercise mat or other soft surface. Extend your arms and place your hands on two medicine balls slightly more than shoulder width apart, keeping your arms straight but not locked and your wrists in line with your shoulders. One at a time, extend your legs behind you until you are balanced on the fronts of your feet, with your legs straight and ankles close together.

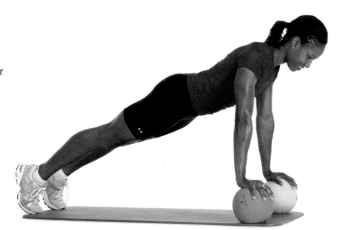

FINISH: Bend your elbows and lower your torso until it is a couple of inches from the medicine balls, with your elbows aligned with your shoulders and your wrists aligned under your elbows. Keep your navel drawn in and maintain a neutral spine. Press back up to the starting position. Perform the recommended number of repetitions.

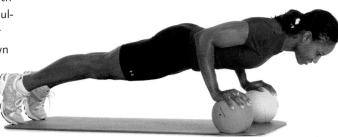

PUSHUP WITH LEG LIFT

START: Kneel on an exercise mat or other soft surface. Extend your arms and place your hands slightly more than shoulder width apart on the mat, keeping your arms straight but not locked and your wrists in line with your shoulders. One at a time, extend your legs behind you until you are balanced on the fronts of your feet, with your legs straight and ankles close together. Raise one leg off the floor.

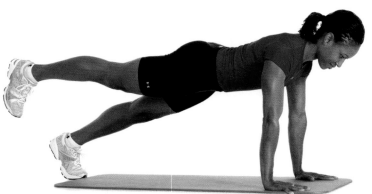

FINISH: Bend your elbows and lower your torso until it is a couple of inches from the floor, with your elbows aligned with your shoulders and your wrists aligned under your elbows. Keep your navel drawn in and maintain a neutral spine. Press back up to the starting position. Perform the recommended number of repetitions then repeat with the other leg raised.

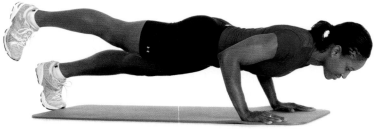

Target muscles: Upper back

BACK BUILDER WITH STABILITY BALL

START: Securely attach exercise tubing to the side of a doorjamb or other sturdy surface at about knee height. Sit on a stability ball with your knees bent and your feet about 12 inches apart.

FINISH: Starting with your arms straight, grasp the handles and pull them in tightly toward your midsection, bending your elbows so they end up slightly behind your torso. At the top of the movement, pull your shoulders back and tense your back muscles for a count or two. Straighten your arms and lean forward slightly. Perform the recommended number of repetitions.

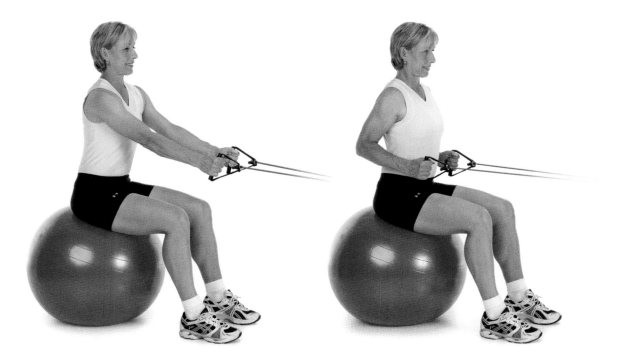

FUNCTIONAL EXERCISES

Functional exercises train your body so that you can perform all sorts of physical tasks you need to do during any given day. Most functional exercises focus on strength and flexibility—two important fitness components required to keep your body in tune for lifting, bending, reaching, turning, and virtually all the moves you need to do.

CRISSCROSS WITH MEDICINE BALL

START: Stand with your body in neutral alignment, holding a medicine ball in front of you. Turn your upper body to the right, bend your knees, and lower your hips as you move the ball down toward the outside of your right foot.

FINISH: Push through your legs and stand up, moving the ball diagonally across your body until your arms are extended above your left shoulder. Return to the starting position, following the same path back across your body. Perform the recommended number of repetitions, then repeat on the other side.

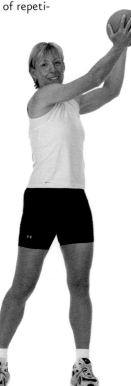
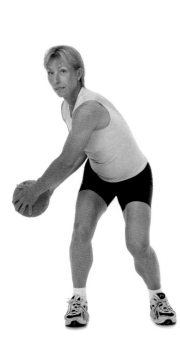

SQUAT TO HIGH LIFT WITH MEDICINE BALL

START: Stand with your feet approximately shoulder width apart, holding a medicine ball in front of you. Keep your feet flat on the floor and your toes pointed slightly outward or in a comfortable position for you.

FINISH: In a slow, controlled movement, move the ball toward the floor by lowering your arms, bending your knees, and lowering your hips as if you're about to sit in a chair. Keep your chest lifted, your core muscles tight, and your eyes focused straight ahead. Slowly return to a standing position, extending through your hips as you raise the ball above your head. Let your chin jut forward and try to keep your rib cage from popping forward. Perform the recommended number of repetitions.

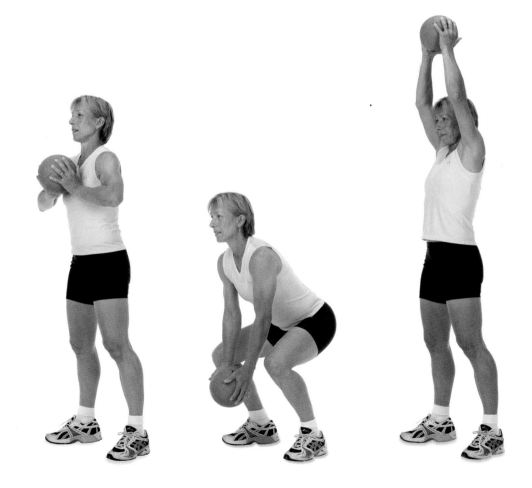

LEG LUNGE WITH XERDISC

START: Place one foot on an Xerdisc and the other about 3 feet behind you. Keep your arms at your sides.

FINISH: Bend your knees until your front thigh is parallel to the floor, then push upward with your feet to return to the starting position. Perform the recommended number of repetitions, then repeat on the other side.

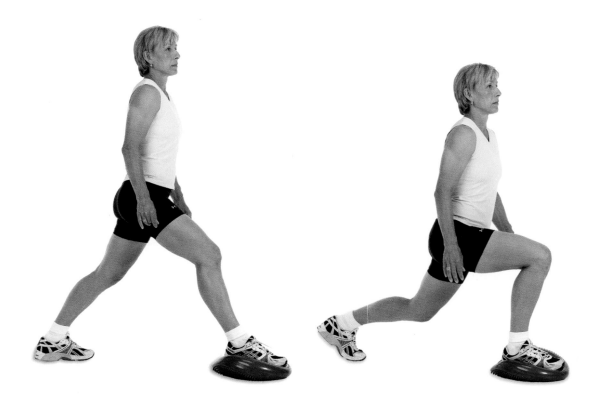

REACH AND ROW WITH XERDISC

START: Wrap exercise tubing around the lower end of a post or anchor it to the lower part of a door-jamb. Grasp the handle in your right hand, step forward with your left leg, and place your left foot squarely on an Xerdisc. Tilt your torso at a 45-degree angle, with your left knee bent in a lunge. Be sure the tension on the tubing lets you maintain neutral alignment without tipping forward.

FINISH: Push back through your legs and body and pull your arm in to your side so your elbow is bent at a 90-degree angle. Squeeze your shoulder blades together and return to the starting position. Perform the recommended number of repetitions, then switch leg positions and repeat with the other arm.

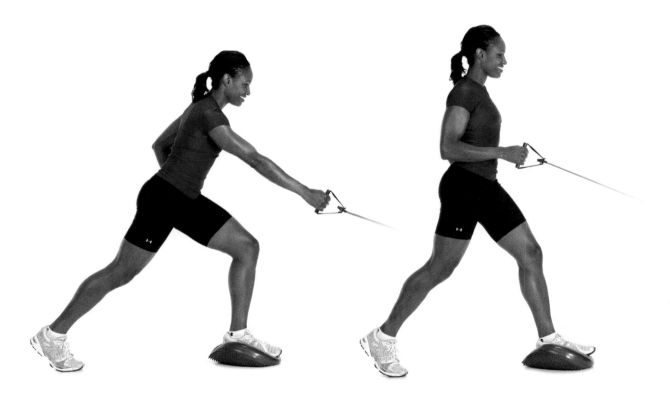

SINGLE-LEG REACH AND ROW

START: Wrap exercise tubing around the lower end of a post or anchor it to the lower part of a doorjamb. Grasp the handle in your right hand and stand on your left leg. Bend at your hips to about a 45-degree angle while maintaining a neutral spine. Be careful not to tip over as you bend forward. Extend your right leg behind you.

FINISH: Pull your arm in to your side so that your elbow is bent at a 90-degree angle. At the same time, draw your right leg in and forward to a bent-knee position in front of you, while simultaneously straightening your back to an erect position. Return to the starting position. Perform the recommended number of repetitions, then repeat with your other arm and leg.

TWISTING LUNGE WITH MEDICINE BALL

START: Stand in a neutral position with your feet hip width apart, holding a medicine ball in front of you. Step forward into a lunge with your right leg and extend the ball in front of you.

FINISH: At the same time, turn your torso and arms to the right, rotating your shoulders without arching your spine. Return to the starting position, following the same path with the ball while pushing through your feet and legs. Perform the recommended number of repetitions, then repeat on the other side.

DUMBBELL SQUAT

START: Stand with your feet about shoulder width apart, holding a dumbbell in each hand.

FINISH: Keeping your head up, slowly bend your knees and lower your hips until your thighs are nearly parallel to the floor. Slowly return to the starting position. Perform the recommended number of repetitions.

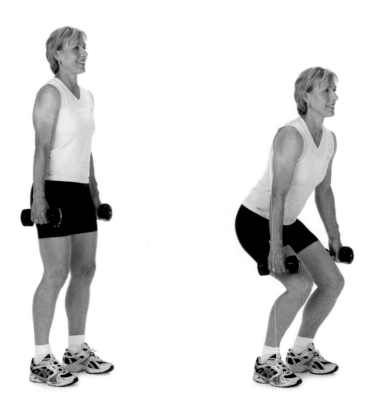

DUMBBELL SQUAT WITH XERDISC

START: Stand on an Xerdisc, holding a dumbbell in each hand.

FINISH: Keeping your head up, slowly bend your knees and lower your hips until your thighs are nearly parallel to the floor. Slowly return to the starting position. Perform the recommended number of repetitions.

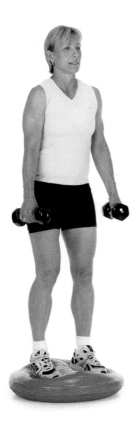
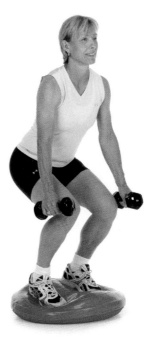

To a great extent, every exercise you do shapes, firms, tightens, and tones some muscle or group of muscles. If what you want from your workout is to isolate and sculpt specific areas of your body, the exercises I've included here will do the trick.

TRICEPS TONER

Target muscles: Backs of upper arms (triceps)

START: Anchor the midpoint of exercise tubing to the top of a doorjamb. Stand facing the door with your feet shoulder width apart and grasp the handles with an underhand grip, with your elbows bent and your upper arms braced against your sides.

FINISH: Press down until your arms are fully extended and your elbows are straight. Slowly return to the starting position. Perform the recommended number of repetitions.

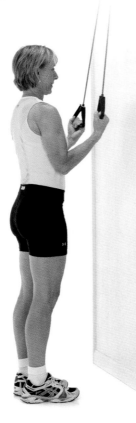 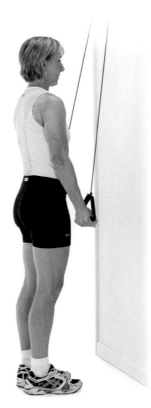

THIGH DOWNSIZER

Target muscles: Upper legs (quadriceps), inner thighs

START: Lie on your side on an exercise mat or soft surface and cross your arms over your chest. For comfort, place your head on a rolled-up towel or other support.

FINISH: Keeping your bottom leg straight, raise your top leg. Slowly return to the starting position. Perform the recommended number of repetitions, then repeat on the other side.

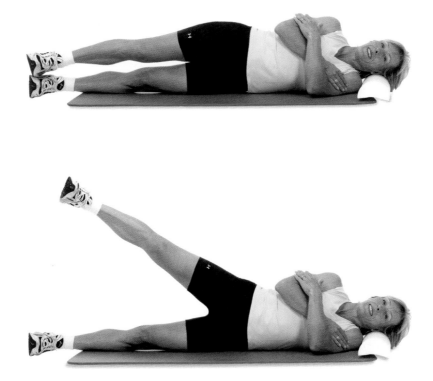

INNER-THIGH SHAPER

Target muscles: Inner thighs

START: Lie on your back on an exercise mat or other soft surface. Bend your knees and place a stability ball between your knees and inner thighs. Keep your arms at your sides.

FINISH: Squeeze the ball between your thighs as hard as you can. Hold for 6 to 10 seconds and release. Perform the recommended number of repetitions.

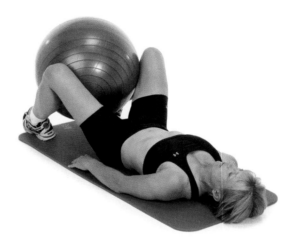

BICEPS CURL

Target muscles: Upper arms (biceps)

START: Stand with your feet shoulder width apart on the midpoint of a length of exercise tubing to create some resistance. Grasp the handles with an underhand grip, keeping your arms at your sides, your chest out, and your shoulders back.

FINISH: Flex your arms at the elbows and pull the handles in an upward arc toward your shoulders, with the palms of your hands facing up and your elbows close to your sides. Pause for a moment to contract your biceps at the peak of the exercise, then return to the starting position. Perform the recommended number of repetitions.

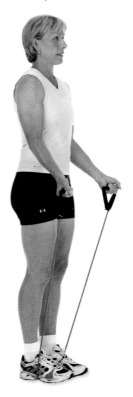 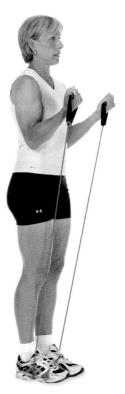

SINGLE-ARM ROW

Target muscles: Upper back (lats), shoulders

START: Step forward with one leg and place your foot on the midpoint of a length of exercise tubing to create some resistance. Grasp one handle and bend forward slightly, keeping your arm extended downward.

FINISH: Pull the handle up and in toward your side. Squeeze your shoulder blades and slowly return to the starting position, keeping your shoulders down throughout the exercise. Perform the recommended number of repetitions, then repeat with the other arm.

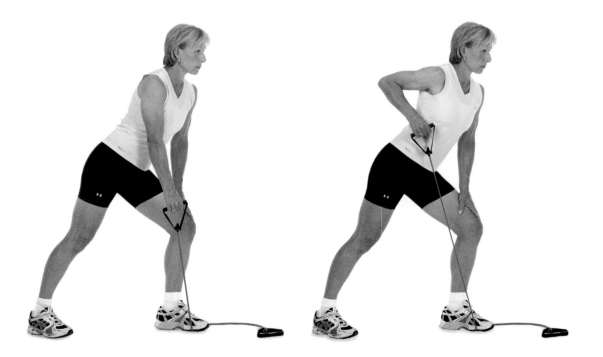

STEPUPS

Target muscles: Legs (quadriceps, hamstrings, and calves)

START: For this exercise, you'll need a platform or bench approximately 6 to 12 inches high. Holding a dumbbell in each hand, step onto the platform, keeping your spine straight and your hips neutral. Be sure to align your knee over your ankle and out past your second toe.

FINISH: Step up with the other leg, making sure your weight is evenly distributed and your knees are straight when both feet are on the platform. Step down and return to the starting position. Continue stepping, then repeat, starting with the other leg. (Or you can do all the reps with one leg, then switch, which is what I like to do.) Perform the recommended number of repetitions. (You may increase the height of the platform as your strength increases.)

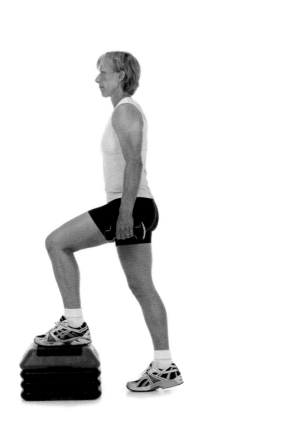
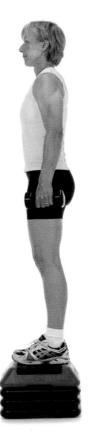

REAR DELT PULL

Target muscles: Backs of shoulders (delts)

START: Stand with your feet shoulder width apart, holding exercise tubing in front of you with a handle in each hand. Extend your arms in front of your chest and move them apart to create resistance.

FINISH: Bend your elbows and pull back on the tubing, concentrating on bringing your shoulder blades together. While pulling, keep your elbows in line with your shoulders. Perform the recommended number of repetitions.

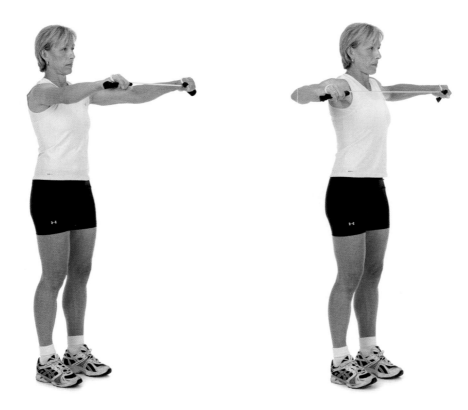

HIP TRIM WITH STABILITY BALL

Target muscles: Hips (gluteals)

START: Lie faceup on a stability ball with your head, neck, and shoulders supported by the ball. Cross your arms over your chest. Bend your knees and position your feet hip width apart, keeping your torso in neutral alignment. Your tailbone should be pulled down slightly and your navel drawn in firmly toward your spine.

FINISH: Push through your feet and raise your hips to neutral position, then return to the starting position. Perform the recommended number of repetitions.

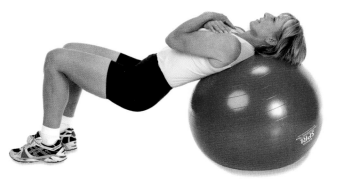

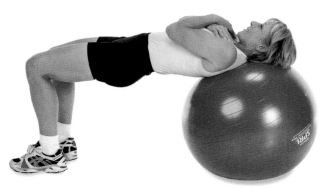

TIP: To increase the intensity of this exercise, hold a light ball or small foam roller between your upper thighs or hold a light dumbbell across your hips.

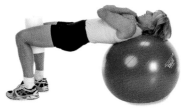

LAT PULLDOWN, BACK

Target muscles: Upper back (lats), chest (pectorals)

START: Hold the handles of exercise tubing and pull it taut. Extend the tubing above your head and stretch it to beyond shoulder width.

FINISH: Pull the tubing down behind your neck until it touches the tops of your shoulder blades. Squeeze your shoulder blades, then slowly return to the starting position. Perform the recommended number of repetitions.

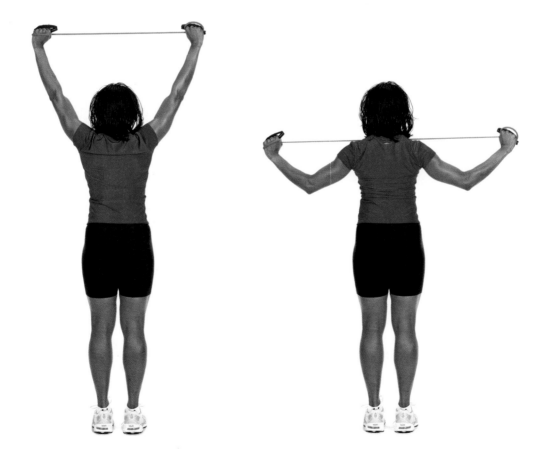

LAT PULLDOWN, FRONT

Target muscles: Upper back (lats), chest (pectorals)

START: Hold the handles of exercise tubing and pull it taut. Extend the tubing above your head and stretch it to beyond shoulder width.

FINISH: Pull the tubing down in front of you until it touches just below the front of your neck. Slowly return to the starting position. Perform the recommended number of repetitions.

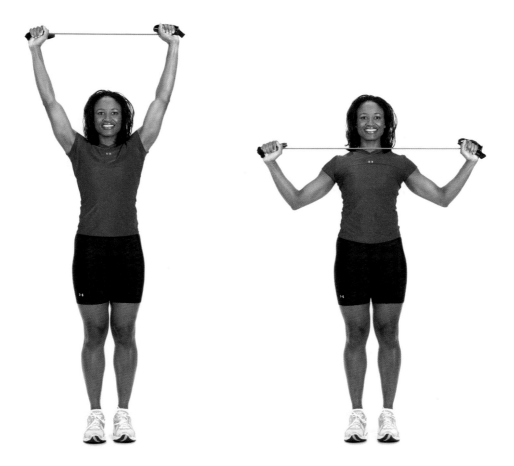

LEG RAISE WITH STABILITY BALL

Target muscles: Buttocks (gluteals) and lower back

START: Lie facedown with your stomach on a stability ball and your hands and feet touching the floor, slightly more than hip width apart. Contract your abs and maintain a neutral position.

FINISH: Lift your legs so they are in line with your body. Contract your gluteal muscles and squeeze your inner thighs together. Release your legs back to slightly more than hip width, then lower them to the floor. Perform the recommended number of repetitions.

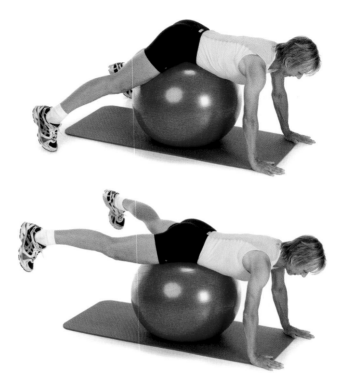

TIP: To increase the intensity of this exercise, wrap exercise tubing around your ankles.

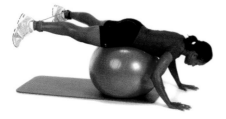

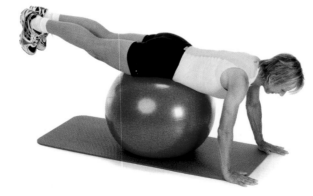

PEC PERFECTER WITH FOAM ROLLER

Target muscles: Upper chest (pectorals), backs of upper arms (triceps)

START: Lie on your back with a foam roller positioned vertically under you and bend your knees. Hold dumbbells directly above your chest, in line with your shoulders.

FINISH: Slowly bend your elbows and lower the dumbbells to the sides of your chest. Try to get a good stretch across your chest, squeezing your pectoral muscles. Press the dumbbells back up to the starting position. Throughout the exercise, be sure to keep the rest of your body in neutral alignment. Perform the recommended number of repetitions.

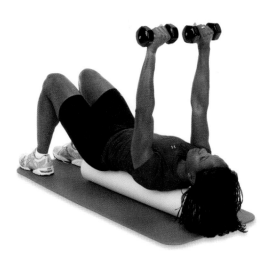

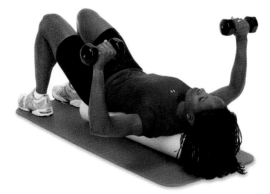

ELEVATED LUNGE

Target muscles: Legs (quadriceps, hamstrings, and calves)

START: Stand with your left foot forward and place your right foot on a platform or bench 6 to 12 inches high. Your front foot should be about 3 feet away from your back foot, with both feet about hip width apart, as shown. Make sure your back knee is aligned over your ankle by moving your front knee out over your second toe. Hold a dumbbell in each hand at your sides.

FINISH: Bend your front knee and lower your hips until your front thigh is nearly parallel to the floor. Pause, then straighten your knee to return to the starting position. Perform the recommended number of repetitions. Switch leg positions and repeat the exercise on the other side.

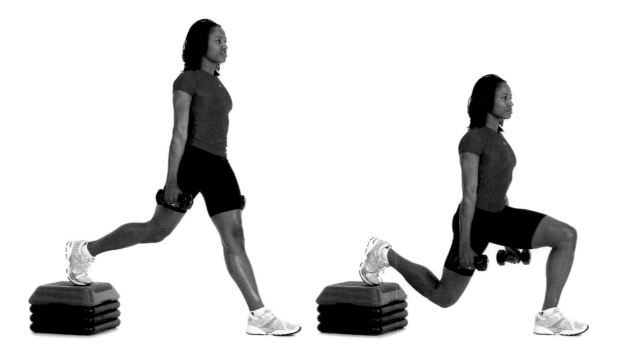

CORRECTIVE EXERCISES FOR POSTURE

The exercises you will do each week include some moves that will help you improve your posture. By strengthening the muscles used to sit, stand, or walk, they help eliminate the stress in your neck and upper back and help you stand tall with confidence. When these muscles are strengthened, a stabilizing "corset" is created that holds them up. You're less likely to hunch over, let your neck droop, or slouch. These exercises are often considered flexibility moves, too, because they act to increase the suppleness of your muscles and joints so your body can move freely, without stiffness or other restrictions.

LYING COBRA

Target: Shoulder and chest posture

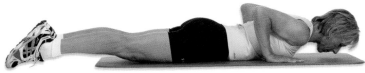

START: Lie on your stomach on an exercise mat or other soft surface with your hands just below your shoulders. Keep your shoulders down and away from your ears and your shoulder blades squeezed together.

FINISH: Gently push into your hands while lifting your chest, keeping your navel pulled inward to support your lower back. Slowly return to the starting position. Perform the recommended number of repetitions.

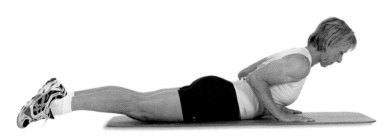

STANDING T

Target: Shoulder and chest posture

START: Stand in a neutral position, holding a dumbbell in each hand with your arms outstretched in front of you.

FINISH: Extend your arms to the sides to form a T shape. Squeeze your shoulder blades together, keeping the palms of your hands facing out. Don't move your chin forward or jut your rib cage out. Return to the starting position. Perform the recommended number of repetitions.

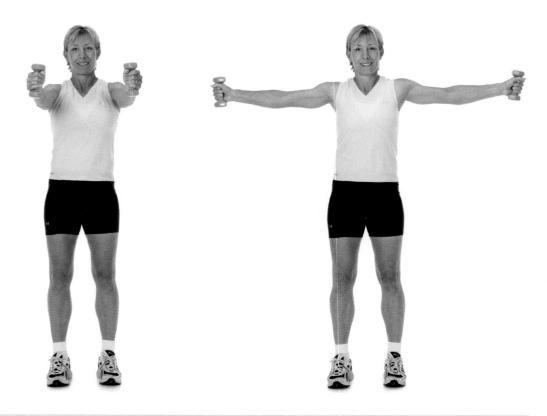

TIP: For an extra challenge, lean forward with your torso at a 45-degree angle as you perform the exercise.

STANDING Y

Target: Upper-body posture

START: Stand in a neutral position, holding a dumbbell in each hand with your arms at your sides.

FINISH: Slowly lift your arms above your head to form a Y shape, with your palms facing each other, and squeeze your shoulder blades together. Don't move your chin forward or jut your rib cage out. Return to the starting position. Perform the recommended number of repetitions.

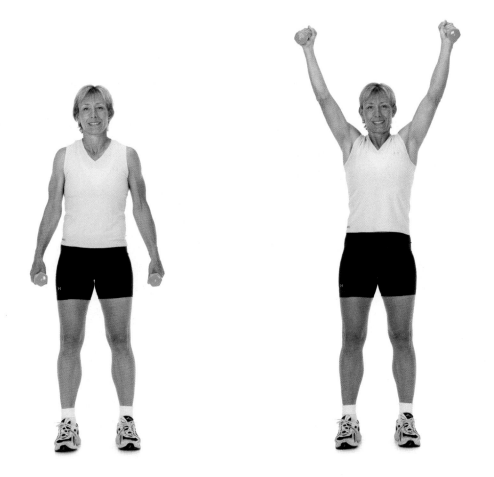

STABILITY BALL Y

Target: Upper-body posture

START: Lie facedown with your upper body on a stability ball and your feet against a wall for support. Hold a dumbbell in each hand with your palms facing each other. While maintaining a neutral spine, slowly lift your arms above your head to form a Y shape.

FINISH: Bend your elbows and lower your arms so they are just in front of you, then raise them to shoulder height while squeezing your shoulder blades together. Return to the starting position. Perform the recommended number of repetitions.

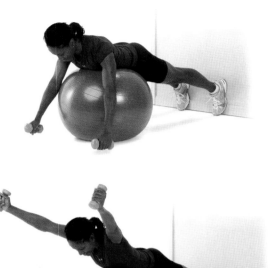

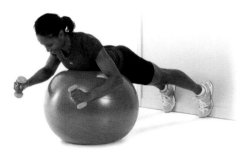

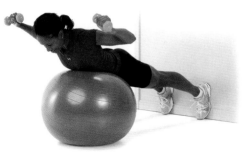

STANDING L

Target: Shoulder and chest posture

START: Stand in a neutral position, with a dumbbell in each hand and your arms bent at 90-degree angles in front of you. Lean forward at a 45-degree angle.

FINISH: Slowly extend your arms to the sides while turning your forearms outward, keeping your elbows close to your sides and squeezing your shoulder blades together. Don't move your chin forward or jut your rib cage out. Return to the starting position. Perform the recommended number of repetitions.

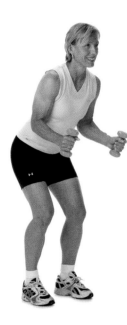
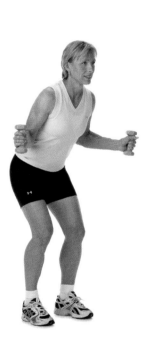

TIP: To make the exercise more challenging, perform the same movements while lying facedown on a stability ball.

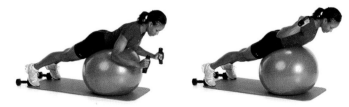

FOAM ROLLER STRETCHES

An important component of a balanced fitness program, flexibility means that your muscles and joints can "give" and move freely. You can increase your flexibility mostly through stretching exercises. A more flexible body helps prevent injury; avoid muscle knots, tightness, and soreness caused by daily activities and exercise; increase your range of motion; promote relaxation; improve your performance and posture; reduce stress; and keep your body feeling youthful and agile.

Although there are lots of flexibility exercises, and most are very good, I like to stretch using a foam roller. These exercises are safe and effective, and they have worked well for me. When using the roller, you'll stretch specific muscles using a slow, gradual, controlled motion to elongate the muscle into its farthest comfortable position, then hold that position for 15 to 30 seconds. This is called static stretching.

Most experts agree that the best time to stretch a muscle is after exercise, when your muscles are warm and blood is circulating freely through your body. Trying to stretch a cold muscle invites injury and damage. What follows is a series of foam roller stretches you can do after your workouts.

IT BAND STRETCH

The IT (iliotibial) band isn't the latest rap or rock group (sorry!). It is a layer of connective tissue that runs down the outside of the leg from the outer side of your hip to below your knee, where it attaches to the outer side of your upper shinbone. When this tissue is injured, your knee can start hurting. This stretch will help keep your IT band flexible and healthy.

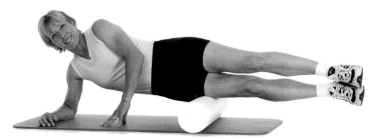

START: Lie on your side with a foam roller under the top of your right thigh. Support your weight with your forearm and keep your torso lifted.

FINISH: Using your arms to propel you, roll from the top of your thigh down the muscled area on the outside of your leg until the roller is right above your knee. Reverse direction to return to the starting position. Repeat three to five times.

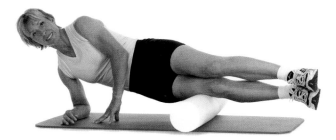

HAMSTRING STRETCH

START: Sit with a foam roller just under your buttocks at the top of your hamstrings, supporting your weight with your hands.

FINISH: Keeping your thighs engaged so your feet don't drag along the floor, roll down your hamstrings until the roller reaches your knees. Reverse direction to return to the starting position. Repeat three to five times. (If you prefer, you can stretch one leg at a time by crossing one foot over the other, which increases the intensity of the stretch.)

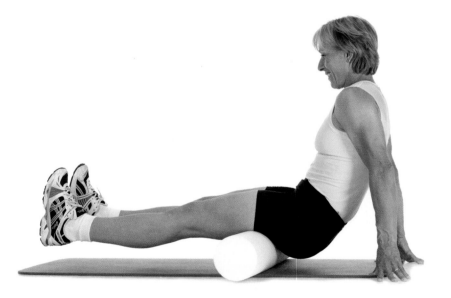

MID-BACK STRETCH

START: Lie on your back with a foam roller under your shoulders and your arms crossed over your chest. Keep your head in neutral alignment or support it with your hands, if necessary.

FINISH: Keeping your hips elevated and your abs tight to support your lower back, roll down from the top of your back to your mid-back. Reverse direction to return to the starting position. Repeat seven or eight times.

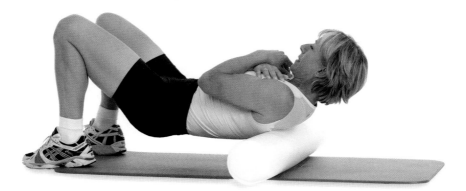

HIP STRETCH

START: Sit with a foam roller under one buttock. Bend your knees and cross one foot over the opposite knee, forming a figure 4 with your legs.

FINISH: Roll along the back of your hip while maintaining the stretch by lightly pulling your knee toward the opposite shoulder. Repeat seven or eight times.

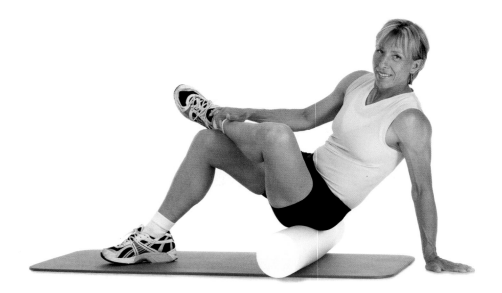

QUAD STRETCH

START: Lie on your stomach with a foam roller under your thighs.

FINISH: Using your arms, pull your body along the floor, allowing the roller to move along the tops of your thighs. Keep your navel drawn in to support your lower back. Repeat three to five times.

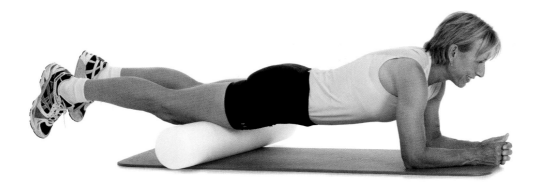

LAT STRETCH

START: Lie on your side with a foam roller just under your armpit at the top of your lat.

FINISH: Gently roll the side of your body along the roller to the end of your rib cage. Raise your torso for more leverage and pressure to massage your lats. Repeat three to five times on each side.

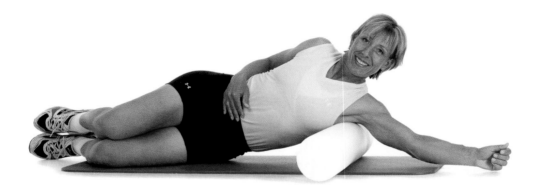

CARDIOVASCULAR EXERCISES

Don't ignore your cardio workouts. Whether it's playing a little one-on-one basketball, jumping rope, or running a few miles a day, I try to do as much cardio as I can throughout the week. It builds up my stamina so much that when I play tennis, I feel like I'm roaring through my matches. To provide an element of fun to the workout, I mix my cardio up, doing a variety of activities. I think the variety helps me stay motivated, plus it gets me in great shape. The way I see it, there's no excuse for getting bored with cardio. Because it's so popular at gyms and fitness centers, there are many activities you can choose from. I've listed some of the different forms of cardio below. Look through them and choose a couple that appeal to you. Try to perform some cardio several days a week.

Cardiovascular Exercise Options

Aerobic dance classes

Basketball, tennis, or soccer

Bicycling

Cross-country skiing or cross-country ski machine

Dance classes

Elliptical trainer

Hiking

Jogging

Jumping rope

Kickboxing classes

Running

Spinning classes

Stair climbing

Stair-stepping machine

Stationary or recumbent bike

Step classes

Swimming

Treadmill

Walking

Water walking or jogging

You'll also want to challenge the power of your cardiovascular system by gradually upping your intensity or, to put it another way, how hard you work out. The greater the intensity of your workouts, the better your health and fitness will be. The best way I've found to challenge your cardiovascular system is by monitoring your level of "perceived exertion." This method was taught to me by one of my trainers, Lisa Austin, and I really prefer it to stopping every now and then and checking my heart rate. Once you get the hang of it, this method will teach you to instinctively know how hard you're working out, in the same way that elite athletes instinctively know the levels of intensity of their workouts without having to check their heart rates.

The following 10-point scale helps you tune in to your level of intensity using subjective descriptions of how the exercise feels as you exert yourself. Get familiar with how it feels to be at levels 4 through 8 because, depending on your conditioning (beginner, intermediate, or advanced), that's the intensity at which I want you to exercise most of the time when you train your cardiovascular system. You can use this scale with any type of cardio exercise, from walking to jogging to bicycling.

Perceived Exertion Scale

1: Very easy. You feel no real effort and are hardly concentrating on the workout. You can talk while exercising. This feels like rest.

2: Easy. This is the way you feel as you move around during daily activities—washing dishes, getting dressed, and so forth. You can still talk while exercising.

3: Moderately easy. This is how you feel when walking around from place to place. In addition, this is how you would typically feel during the warmup and cooldown phases of exercise. Your breathing begins to become elevated, but only slightly.

4: Moderate. You are right below half of your maximum effort, with your breathing becoming more elevated.

5: Moderately hard. This is how you would feel if you took a brisk walk. It feels like a light workout during which you might say to yourself, "I'm getting a good workout, but I'm not killing myself." Your breathing is more elevated.

6: Still moderately hard. This is how you would feel if you picked up the pace of your brisk walk. Your breathing is deeper, and it's a little harder to carry on a conversation. You may start to feel some fatigue, but this is still a level of effort you feel you can maintain for a while.

7: A little difficult. You have now reached the level of vigorous exercise. You do feel a little more tired, and your breathing is quite deep. You can still carry on a conversation, but it requires more effort. You're aware, too, that your heart is pumping hard. Don't stop now!

8: Difficult. This level feels like a very vigorous, very strenuous effort. Your breathing is very deep, and it's difficult to carry on a conversation. Your body is working very hard; maintaining this level for at least 20 minutes will help you start to burn fat and condition your heart and lungs.

9: Very difficult. You are surely pushing yourself at a very high level of effort, and you may start to feel very fatigued. Your breathing is labored, and conversation would require too much effort. Most elite athletes train at this level.

10: Maximum difficulty. This level requires all-out intensity that cannot be maintained very long at all. Most exercise experts say there is no value in reaching this level because it can leave you drained and offers no additional cardiovascular benefits.

FINDING YOUR LEVEL

The exercise routines that follow are set up for beginner, intermediate, and advanced exercisers. Here's how to tell where you fit.

Beginner

You're a brand-new exerciser, with little or no experience in fitness or in any particular movement skills, or you may have exercise experience, but your workouts are few and far between.

Intermediate

You exercise regularly, perhaps several times a week. What's more, you have a good working knowledge of various types of exercises.

Advanced

You have exercised for several years, always challenging yourself to higher intensities, and would be considered to be in good shape. You may also be an athlete who competes regularly.

If you've determined that you're a beginner or intermediate, one of your goals should be to work up to the advanced routine. No matter where you start, once your routine becomes less challenging, it's time to progress to the next level. Constantly challenge yourself to do more, and you'll get more out of your body—and your life.

BEGINNER: *Weeks 1 and 2*

EXERCISE	FUNCTION/BODY PART	WEEK 1 GOAL	WEEK 2 GOAL
Tummy Tuck	Core	10–12 reps, 1 set, 3 times a week	10–12 reps, 1 set, 3 times a week
Lying Cobra	Shoulder and chest posture	10–12 reps, 1 set, 3 times a week	10–12 reps, 1 set, 3 times a week
Bun Burner	Core	10–12 reps, 1 set, 3 times a week	10–12 reps, 1 set, 3 times a week
Wall Squat with Stability Ball or Dumbbell Squat	Lower-body strength/core	10–12 reps, 1 set, 3 times a week	10–12 reps, 1 set, 3 times a week
Bent-Knee Pushup	Upper-body strength/triceps	10–12 reps, 1 set, 3 times a week	10–12 reps, 1 set, 3 times a week
Biceps Curl	Body shaping/arms	10–12 reps, 1 set, 3 times a week	10–12 reps, 1 set, 3 times a week
Thigh Downsizer	Body shaping/legs	10–12 reps, 1 set, 3 times a week	10–12 reps, 1 set, 3 times a week
Lat Pulldown, Front, or Lat Pulldown, Back	Body shaping/upper back, chest	10–12 reps, 1 set, 3 times a week	10–12 reps, 1 set, 3 times a week
Squat to High Lift with Medicine Ball	Functional movement	10–12 reps, 1 set, 3 times a week	10–12 reps, 1 set, 3 times a week
Foam roller stretch series	Flexibility	3–5 times a week	3–5 times a week
Cardio*	Cardiovascular health	Perceived exertion = 4–5 for 15 minutes, 3 times a week	Perceived exertion = 5–6 for 15–20 minutes, 3 times a week

* Each cardio session should begin and end with 5 to 10 minutes of light cardiovascular activity at a perceived exertion of 2 to 3.

BEGINNER: *Weeks 3 and 4*

EXERCISE	FUNCTION/BODY PART	WEEK 3 GOAL	WEEK 4 GOAL
Tummy Tuck with Stability Ball	Core	12–15 reps, 2 sets, 3 times a week	12–15 reps, 2 sets, 3 times a week
Bun Burner with Xerdisc	Core	12–15 reps, 2 sets, 3 times a week	12–15 reps, 2 sets, 3 times a week
Standing T	Shoulder and chest posture	12–15 reps, 2 sets, 3 times a week	12–15 reps, 2 sets, 3 times a week
Torso Toner	Core	12–15 reps, 2 sets, 3 times a week	12–15 reps, 2 sets, 3 times a week
Split-Stance Squat with Stability Ball	Lower-body strength/legs	12–15 reps, 2 sets, 3 times a week	12–15 reps, 2 sets, 3 times a week
Bent-Knee Pushup on Unstable Surface	Upper-body strength/triceps	12–15 reps, 2 sets, 3 times a week	12–15 reps, 2 sets, 3 times a week
Back Builder with Stability Ball	Upper-body strength/back	12–15 reps, 2 sets, 3 times a week	12–15 reps, 2 sets, 3 times a week
Biceps Curl	Body shaping/arms	12–15 reps, 2 sets, 3 times a week	12–15 reps, 2 sets, 3 times a week
Inner-Thigh Shaper	Body shaping/legs	12–15 reps, 2 sets, 3 times a week	12–15 reps, 2 sets, 3 times a week
Pec Perfecter with Foam Roller	Body shaping/chest, triceps	12–15 reps, 2 sets, 3 times a week	12–15 reps, 2 sets, 3 times a week
Crisscross with Medicine Ball	Functional movement	12–15 reps, 2 sets, 3 times a week	12–15 reps, 2 sets, 3 times a week
Foam roller stretch series	Flexibility	3–5 times a week	3–5 times a week
Cardio*	Cardiovascular health	Perceived exertion = 5–6 for 20 minutes, 3 times a week	Perceived exertion = 5–6 for 20 minutes, 3 times a week

* Each cardio session should begin and end with 5 to 10 minutes of light cardiovascular activity at a perceived exertion of 2 to 3.

INTERMEDIATE: *Weeks 1 and 2*

EXERCISE	FUNCTION/BODY PART	WEEK 1 GOAL	WEEK 2 GOAL
Waist Whittler	Core	10–12 reps, 2 sets, 3 times a week	10–12 reps, 2 sets, 3 times a week
Standing Y	Shoulder and chest posture	10–12 reps, 2 sets, 3 times a week	10–12 reps, 2 sets, 3 times a week
"Dead Bug" Heel Tap with Foam Roller	Core	10–12 reps, 2 sets, 3 times a week	10–12 reps, 2 sets, 3 times a week
Dumbbell Squat with Xerdisc	Lower-body strength/legs	10–12 reps, 2 sets, 3 times a week	10–12 reps, 2 sets, 3 times a week
Bent-Knee Pushup on Unstable Surface	Upper-body strength/triceps	10–12 reps, 2 sets, 3 times a week	10–12 reps, 2 sets, 3 times a week
Biceps Curl	Body shaping/biceps	10–12 reps, 2 sets, 3 times a week	10–12 reps, 2 sets, 3 times a week
Single-Arm Row	Body shaping/back	10–12 reps, 2 sets, 3 times a week	10–12 reps, 2 sets, 3 times a week
Stepups	Body shaping/legs	10–12 reps, 2 sets, 3 times a week	10–12 reps, 2 sets, 3 times a week
Leg Lunge with Xerdisc or Elevated Lunge	Functional movement	10–12 reps, 2 sets, 3 times a week	10–12 reps, 2 sets, 3 times a week
Foam roller stretch series	Flexibility	3–5 times a week	3–5 times a week
Cardio*	Cardiovascular health	Perceived exertion = 6–7 for 20–25 minutes, 4 times a week	Perceived exertion = 6–7 for 20–25 minutes, 4 times a week

* Each cardio session should begin and end with 5 to 10 minutes of light cardiovascular activity at a perceived exertion of 2 to 3.

INTERMEDIATE: *Weeks 3 and 4*

EXERCISE	FUNCTION/BODY PART	WEEK 3 GOAL	WEEK 4 GOAL
Waist Whittler	Core	12–15 reps, 2 sets, 3 times a week	12–15 reps, 2 sets, 3 times a week
Bun Burner with Leg Lift on Xerdisc	Core	12–15 reps, 2 sets, 3 times a week	12–15 reps, 2 sets, 3 times a week
Standing L	Shoulder and chest posture	12–15 reps, 2 sets, 3 times a week	12–15 reps, 2 sets, 3 times a week
"Dead Bug" Heel Tap with Foam Roller	Core	12–15 reps, 2 sets, 3 times a week	12–15 reps, 2 sets, 3 times a week
Dumbbell Squat with Xerdisc	Lower-body strength/legs	12–15 reps, 2 sets, 3 times a week	12–15 reps, 2 sets, 3 times a week
Pushup	Upper-body strength/triceps	12–15 reps, 2 sets, 3 times a week	12–15 reps, 2 sets, 3 times a week
Biceps Curl	Body shaping/biceps	12–15 reps, 2 sets, 3 times a week	12–15 reps, 2 sets, 3 times a week
Rear Delt Pull	Body shaping/shoulders, arms	12–15 reps, 2 sets, 3 times a week	12–15 reps, 2 sets, 3 times a week
Waist Whittler on Unstable Surface	Body shaping/core, hips, gluteals	12–15 reps, 2 sets, 3 times a week	12–15 reps, 2 sets, 3 times a week
Reach and Row with Xerdisc	Functional movement	12–15 reps, 2 sets, 3 times a week	12–15 reps, 2 sets, 3 times a week
Foam roller stretch series	Flexibility	3–5 times a week	3–5 times a week
Cardio*	Cardiovascular health	Perceived exertion = 6–7 for 20–25 minutes, 4 times a week	Perceived exertion = 6–7 for 25–30 minutes, 4 times a week

* Each cardio session should begin and end with 5 to 10 minutes of light cardiovascular activity at a perceived exertion of 2 to 3.

ADVANCED: *Weeks 1 and 2*

EXERCISE	FUNCTION/BODY PART	WEEK 1 GOAL	WEEK 2 GOAL
Waist Whittler	Core	12–15 reps, 2 sets, 3 times a week	12–15 reps, 2 sets, 3 times a week
Stability Ball Y	Shoulder and chest posture	12–15 reps, 2 sets, 3 times a week	12–15 reps, 2 sets, 3 times a week
Bun Burner	Core	12–15 reps, 2 sets, 3 times a week	12–15 reps, 2 sets, 3 times a week
Single-Leg Squat	Lower-body strength/legs	12–15 reps, 2 sets, 3 times a week	12–15 reps, 2 sets, 3 times a week
Pushup with Medicine Balls	Upper-body strength/ triceps	12–15 reps, 2 sets, 3 times a week	12–15 reps, 2 sets, 3 times a week
Biceps Curl	Body shaping/ biceps	12–15 reps, 2 sets, 3 times a week	12–15 reps, 2 sets, 3 times a week
Triceps Toner	Body shaping/ triceps	12–15 reps, 2 sets, 3 times a week	12–15 reps, 2 sets, 3 times a week
Lat Pulldown, Back	Body shaping/ upper back, chest	12–15 reps, 2 sets, 3 times a week	12–15 reps, 2 sets, 3 times a week
Leg Raise with Stability Ball	Body shaping/lower back, hips, buttocks, inner thighs	12–15 reps, 2 sets, 3 times a week	12–15 reps, 2 sets, 3 times a week
Reach and Row with Xerdisc or Single-Leg Reach and Row	Functional movement	12–15 reps, 2 sets, 3 times a week	12–15 reps, 2 sets, 3 times a week
Foam roller stretch series	Flexibility	3–5 times a week	3–5 times a week
Cardio*	Cardiovascular health	Perceived exertion = 7–8 for 30–35 minutes, 5 times a week	Perceived exertion = 7–8 for 30–35 minutes, 5 times a week

* Each cardio session should begin and end with 5 to 10 minutes of light cardiovascular activity at a perceived exertion of 2 to 3.

ADVANCED: *Weeks 3 and 4*

EXERCISE	FUNCTION/BODY PART	WEEK 3 GOAL	WEEK 4 GOAL
Twist or Twist Up	Core	12–15 reps, 3 sets, 3 times a week	12–15 reps, 3 sets, 3 times a week
Core Cruncher with Stability Ball	Core	12–15 reps, 3 sets, 3 times a week	12–15 reps, 3 sets, 3 times a week
Tummy Tightener with Foam Roller	Core	12–15 reps, 3 sets, 3 times a week	12–15 reps, 3 sets, 3 times a week
Single-Leg Squat with Xerdisc	Lower-body strength/legs	12–15 reps, 3 sets, 3 times a week	12–15 reps, 3 sets, 3 times a week
Pushup with Leg Lift	Upper-body strength/ triceps	12–15 reps, 3 sets, 3 times a week	12–15 reps, 3 sets, 3 times a week
Biceps Curl	Body shaping/biceps	12–15 reps, 3 sets, 3 times a week	12–15 reps, 3 sets, 3 times a week
Triceps Toner	Body shaping/triceps	12–15 reps, 3 sets, 3 times a week	12–15 reps, 3 sets, 3 times a week
Pec Perfecter with Foam Roller	Body shaping/chest	12–15 reps, 3 sets, 3 times a week	12–15 reps, 3 sets, 3 times a week
Elevated Lunge	Body shaping/legs	12–15 reps, 3 sets, 3 times a week	12–15 reps, 3 sets, 3 times a week
Twisting Lunge with Medicine Ball	Functional movement	12–15 reps, 3 sets, 3 times a week	12–15 reps, 3 sets, 3 times a week
Foam roller stretch series	Flexibility	3–5 times a week	3–5 times a week
Cardio*	Cardiovascular health	Perceived exertion = 8 for 30–35 minutes, 5–6 times a week	Perceived exertion = 8 for 30–35 minutes, 5–6 times a week

* Each cardio session should begin and end with 5 to 10 minutes of light cardiovascular activity at a perceived exertion of 2 to 3.

WILL THESE WORKOUTS WORK FOREVER?

Yes, but if you want ongoing improvement after the first month, you need to advance your training. If you are a beginner, for example, you can advance to the intermediate level and later to the advanced workout; if you're an intermediate, you can move up to the advanced level. If you are already an experienced exerciser, you can add more of the advanced moves into your routine or use greater resistance with weights or exercise tubing.

As you progress, you must stay attuned to your body. It is wise; it will tell you what you should do and what you shouldn't do. When an exercise feels too easy, that's your body telling you it's time to work harder on that exercise.

When I do cardio workouts, since I prefer speed over endurance, I do an aerobic workout warmup for 10 minutes, then do sprints on the bike, the treadmill, or even a stair-stepper. I might do 30 sprints of going all out for 10 to 15 seconds and resting for 30 seconds in between, or I might do 10 semi-sprints of 1 minute each with breaks of $1\frac{1}{2}$ minutes. Sometimes I base my rest periods on my heart rate recovery. For the shorter sprints, I wait until my heart rate slows to 150 beats per minute before beginning again, and for the longer ones, I wait until it slows to 120. See what works for you, but I find these kinds of cardio workouts—often called interval training—exhilarating and more interesting than just staying at the same speed for 30 minutes.

Make your workouts a challenge. Keep track of what you do, and how much, so you can compare your progress to previous workouts. Mix it up, too, especially by doing different forms of cardio as I do. This will help shock your body into even greater improvement and will keep your workouts interesting. Just keep at it, enjoy yourself, and you will become the best you've ever been.

MY PARTING SHOT

*I hope, when I stop, people will think
that somehow I mattered.*

Throughout this book, I have tried to share my thoughts with you. I don't expect overnight success, and neither should you. But my hope is to encourage you to keep on trying. I really like the old saying, "If at first you don't succeed, try, try again." Just look at me. In 2000, they told me I shouldn't go back and play tennis again—I was too old, they were too good—basically saying I didn't have what it takes anymore. If I had listened to them, I would not have won two more Grand Slam titles.

As long as you believe in yourself, the sky is the limit. Or maybe not even that—just look at Eileen Collins, the space shuttle commander. You never know how far you can go unless you attempt to get there. The key is to believe in yourself, believe that it's possible, and believe that you can do it.

I believe everyone has the power to make things happen, and I encourage everyone to share their successes and failures with me so we can all help one another. Do yourself a favor—don't beat yourself up if at first you don't succeed. Realize that those who achieved great things, both in the present and the past, have failed at one time or another, but they continued to try—and obviously, they succeeded. Even Michelangelo redid his work in the Sistine Chapel because he didn't like the results the first time around.

People have been asking me for a long time what I will do when my career is over. I don't worry about that, really, because there are many things I want to do with my life. I realize I won't be able to play competitively forever, but I plan to keep playing as long as my heart says to keep going, providing my body holds up.

I've been playing so many more years than I expected to, anyway. Each time I'm asked if this is my last tournament, I say, "I don't know, but I don't think so." I'm not worried about it.

I have to admit that there is still magic in walking through a crowd on the way to the court, but the best is when little kids shout, "Go Martina!"—yet another generation of fans I am lucky to play in front of these days. People like my spirit, I think. It transcends all the usual barriers. My sexuality doesn't matter, nor does where I'm from, that I'm left-handed, or that I'm a woman. People appreciate who I am when I'm playing tennis. That's what it's all about.

I love the fans. They keep me going. A few years ago, while getting ready to play at Eastbourne, I spotted an elderly woman with a walking support who had come to see me play. How honored and moved I was that someone would make such an effort to come to my match. The fans are amazing. It's still fun to go out there and play for them, to hear them hoot and holler and get all excited because they saw me hit a great shot and they can't wait to try it themselves the next time they play.

Once I do say good-bye to professional ten-nis, I'll be able to devote a lot more time to some of my favorite causes—helping to preserve nature and wildlife, cleaning up the environment, really getting involved in helping get equal—not special—rights for gays and lesbians, and just trying to make the world better in some way. A lot of times I'm asked if I will get involved in politics—you know, like Arnold Schwarzenegger did. If I can make a difference, sure, I might go that route, but being an activist is more up my alley. You can take a stand and say exactly what you want without having to worry about hurting someone's feelings or playing games. I'm not much of a politician or diplomat, though. I just sort of blurt out whatever comes into my head, which doesn't work that well in politics.

I will stay involved in tennis, of course. It has given me a fantastic life and opportunities for my family and friends. I want to give back to tennis because I haven't given as much to it as it has given to me. One project in the works is the Martina Navratilova Tennis Academy for children of all ages, incomes, and nationalities who want to become better players. I hope to bring together all the great coaches and trainers I've had, give the kids scholarships, and let them experience the invaluable instruction and mentoring that I have benefited from and am so grateful for.

I'm working to establish the academy in Sarasota, Florida, where I live. I like it there. It's quiet and peaceful; people are friendly. The area abounds in natural beauty, with its crushed-shell beaches and mangrove-ringed, manatee-populated inland waterways. After being on tour, I can't wait to get home, see my dogs, run on the beach, jump in my little motorboat with some friends, and cruise up and down those waterways.

Priorities change as you get older and, hopefully, wiser. It was all tennis and winning earlier in my career, and there's nothing wrong with that. But today, I live to make a difference in people's lives. Once I heard from a young lesbian who felt so alone with her sexuality that she couldn't see past tomorrow and was thus on the brink of committing suicide. Then she saw an interview with me on TV and saw how I live with pride and dignity, not hiding anything. My story made her feel better about who she was, and her thoughts of suicide disappeared. You never know whose life you will touch with your own.

My hope is that this book has touched your life in a positive way as well. I have talked to you about the restorative qualities of food, fitness, and a healthy lifestyle, mostly through my own experiences. I have shared how I manage to stay at my best and give my best effort to everything I do. I know that whatever energy I bring to the world comes first from the quality of the food I put in my body. The secret of harnessing that energy is to eat fresh, whole, organic foods in as natural a state as possible and as often as possible. When you start there, all the rest—exercise, stress reduction, physical stamina, mental and emotional health—will flow naturally to give you the strength you need to carry on.

Perhaps I have introduced you to some new ideas through these six steps. If so, don't be afraid to try what is new or different to you. I have never believed in playing it safe on the tennis court, and I still don't. Some of the best tennis I've ever played has happened when I moved out of my comfort zone and played a brave and confident game—and what fun it was!

Similarly, I have never believed in playing it safe in life. Otherwise, I would still be living in the Czech Republic, and I would never have had the opportunity to get the most out of myself on the tennis court.

I like to create. I like to make things happen. In other words, I come to the net. That is where all the fun happens. I try to find an opening, then I go for it. This is how I play tennis; this is how I live my life.

My advice: Look for the openings, and even if you don't "win," you will have a lot of fun trying. There are opportunities for victory in your life. Be adventurous. Make the necessary changes; don't be afraid of them and what will happen. Once you try something different, you'll realize how easy it really was to change. Who knows? You may just turn your life around for the better and experience a quality of life you never knew existed.

I have discussed the idea of shaping your self in terms of personal fitness. Yes, the shape of your self is that, but it also transcends it. Living the idea takes into account what you do with the rest of your life, too—how you share your talents, treasures, and time. If you take proper care of yourself, you can do it for others. As I've said—in the long run, it's what you leave behind that counts. And I don't mean the size of an inheritance but rather how you affected those around you, how many people's or other creatures' lives you touched in a positive way. I truly think leaving this world a better place than you found it is what gives you a true sense of accomplishment about what you're doing in life. It gives your life purpose and meaning and ultimately shapes it. Take the energy you bring to the world and use it in a positive way. Volunteer. Give some money to a great charity. Do your part. If more people did that, we would have a lot fewer problems.

Remember this: You are the benchmark of your success—you define it. Don't let anyone else define it because if you do, you will fail. Appreciate those who support you and challenge those who don't.

Let me leave you with this parting shot. As you strive to change, caring for yourself, doing for others, and becoming better than you are right now, know that you will have good days and bad days. Nothing in life is ever a straight climb to the mountaintop. There are backsliding, slipping on rocks, and days when you feel that you can't take another step. The pain and frustration of the bad days will pass. Life goes on, and the sun comes up in the morn-

ing. What is important is that you keep getting up, keep going in the direction of your dreams and goals, and keep trying to elevate yourself, no matter what the obstacle. You will get there as long as you let go of the need to be perfect and strive for excellence in every choice you make.

As you move along the path, please visit me at www.martinanavratilova.com to continue to receive current updates, new topics, new recipes, and product testing and information. This site will also be a place where you can share your individual experience with other readers, gain support when facing tough obstacles, and address the many questions that arise along the way.

I know you can win at whatever you set out to do. The rest of your life is in front of you, so give it your best shot. Let today be the beginning of a fresh start. And, if it makes any difference, know that I will be pulling for you all the way, cheering you on, encouraging you and saying, "Come on, you can do it. Just hit the darn ball and go for it." And when in doubt, go to the net!

INDEX

Underscored page references indicate boxed text and tables. **Boldface** references indicate photographs.

Gretzky, Wayne, 73
Grocery shopping, 26
Guacamole
    Guacamole Wraps, 121

H

Haas, Robert, 33
Habitual patterns, breaking, 1, 6
Hamstring stretch, 200, **200**
Happiness, 100
Health and Fitness Inventory, 9, 10–11
Hepburn, Katharine, xx, 20
Hip stretch, 202, **202**
Hip trim with stability ball, 187, **187**
Hormones
    diet for balancing, 47
    in meats, avoiding, 68
How to Think Like Leonardo da Vinci (Gelb), 13
Huber, Liezel, 98

I

Iliotibial band. *See* IT band; IT band stretch
Injuries, in athletes, 84–85, 87
Inner-thigh shaper, 182, **182**
Insecticides, natural, 72
Insulin resistance, 47
Intermediate-level exerciser, 207
    exercise routines for, 210–11
Irradiated foods, 48
IT band, 81, 199
IT band stretch, 199, **199**

J

Jet lag, 96
Jordan, Michael, 23, 72–73
Journaling, 20–23, 85, 93

Juicers
    alternatives to, 52
    recommended, 53
Juices, fresh
    alternatives to, 53
    Apple-Veggie Juice, 124
    benefits of, 52, 53
    Cabbage Cooler, 135
    Carrot-Beet Juice, 123
    Carrot Juice, 118
    cautions about, 54
    Cucumber Cocktail, 132
    for energy, 93
    Gingery Juice, 138
    guidelines for drinking, 54, 115
    Martina's 8, 120
    Mock Wine, 137
    Salad in a Glass, 128
    Spicy Juice, 134
    variety of, 54

K

Kardon, Craig, 21
King, Billie Jean, 14, 21, 41, 75, 100

L

Labels, food
    Certified Organic, 65
    reading, 69
Lat pulldown, back, 188, **188**
Lat pulldown, front, 189, **189**
Lat stretch, 204, **204**
Laundry products, organic, 72
Laver, Rod, 17, 18
Lawn and garden products, organic, 72
Leg lunge with Xerdisc, 174, **174**
Leg raise with stability ball, 190, **190**

early ambitions of, 17–18
fitness formula of, xi–xii
focus of, 23–24
functional fitness of, 74, 76
future plans of, 216–17
journaling by, 20–21, 22
on making lifestyle changes, xix–xxi
nutritional evolution of, 46–48
as Olympic athlete, xviii–xix
ongoing health improvements in, xiii
parting advice of, 217–18
retirement of, xvii–xviii
stressful experiences of, 99–100
on succeeding, 215–16
support system of
in childhood, 31–32
in professional career, 32–33
on teamwork, 33–35
wake-up calls of, 28
weight fluctuations of, xvi–xvii
Wimbledon wins of, 20, 21, 27
Negative people, dealing with, 36–39
Neutral spine or alignment, 77, 148
Newberry, Janet, 27
Nut milks, 111
Almond Milk, 118
blender-made, 52
nutrients in, 54, 115
Raspberry–Almond Milk Smoothie,
126
Nutritional supplements, 56
Nutritionist, 41
Nutrition plan. *See also* Diet(s)
benefits of, xiii, 7, 9, 108
foods in
dairy foods and substitutes,
111–12
fruits, 110
healthy fats, 113–14
low-fat proteins, 112–13
power carbs, 110–11
vegetables, 108–9

guidelines for, 114–15
serving sizes in, 114
variety of foods in, 108
Nuts
calcium in, 115
Energy Balls, 130

O

Oatmeal
Energy Balls, 130
Obesity and overweight
in America vs. other countries, 4
causes of, 108
in children and adults, xv
effects of, 4, 11–12
Omega-3 fatty acids, 51, 54, 62
Omelet
Vegetable and Cheese Omelet, 118
Onions
Vegetable and Cheese Omelet, 118
Vegetable Frittata, 144
Vegetable Stir-Fry, 143
Oranges
Spicy Juice, 134
Organic environment, 7, 71–72
Organic foods, 59–60
benefits of, 11
better taste of, 62
certification of, 65
definition of, 7, 61
nutrients in, 62
reasons for eating, 62–64
restaurants serving, 65
sources of, 7, 64–65, 66–67
Organic milk, 62
Ortega, Stefan, 41, 43–44
Overeating, preventing, 115
Overton, Wendy, xvi
Overtraining, 83
Overweight. *See* Obesity and overweight

P

Paes, Leander, xviii, 16–17
Pancakes
    Potato Pancakes, 144
Parfait
    Berry Parfait, 135
Parma, George, 18
Parties, controlling eating at, 19, 26
Pasta
    Pasta Genovese with Pesto Sauce,
      126
    Pasta Primavera, 139
    recommended, 111
    Tofu Roll-Ups, 129
    whole wheat, 69
Paterno, Joe, 25
Peaches
    Peach Tart, 131
Pears
    Honey-Baked Pears, 121
    Spicy Juice, 134
Pec perfecter with foam roller, 191,
    191
Peppers, bell
    Martina's 8, 120
    Vegetable Frittata, 144
Perceived exertion scale, in cardiovascular
    exercise, 205–6
Perfection, 14, 15
Performance-enhancing substances, 56
Personal care products, organic, 71
Personal trainer, 41, 42
Pesticides
    adverse effects of, 63
    levels of, in fruits and vegetables, 64
    residues of, 62–63, 65
Pesto
    Easy Italian Sub, 140
    Pasta Genovese with Pesto Sauce,
      126
Pets, for stress reduction, 102

Physical activity. *See* Exercise
Portion control, 59
    estimating serving sizes for, 116–17
    in restaurants, 55
Positive people, for support system,
    35–36
Post-exercise snacks, 94–95
Posture awareness, 76–77. *See also* Corrective
    exercises for posture
Potatoes
    Potato Pancakes, 144
Poultry, as protein source, 113
Power carbs, 110–11
    serving sizes of, 116–17
Preparation, importance of, 25–26
Preservatives, food, 11, 69
Prioritizing, for stress reduction, 102
Processed foods, problems with, 11, 47, 48,
    93
Procrastination, 13
Protein
    animal sources of, 112, 113
    importance of, 112
    for post-exercise snacks, 94–95
    serving sizes of, 117
    vegetarian sources of, 112
Pudding
    Tropical Pudding, 143
Pumpkin seeds, omega-3 fatty acids in, 51
Pushup(s), 168, **168**
    bent-knee pushup, 166, **166**
    bent-knee pushup on unstable surface, 167,
      167
    pushup with leg lift, 170, **170**
    pushup with medicine balls, 169, **169**
Pushup with leg lift, 170, **170**
Pushup with medicine balls, 169, **169**

Q

Quad stretch, 203, **203**

Water *(cont.)*
    for preventing fatigue, 93–94
    for rehydration after exercise, 95
    tap, contaminants in, 57
Water filtration systems, 57
Weight loss
    from healthy diet, <u>59</u>
    maintaining focus for, 24
    number of servings for, 114
    worry affecting, 24
Weight-loss diets, problems with, 49
Weight machines, 78
White noise, for falling asleep, 97
Whole grains, 69, 115
    nutrients in, <u>11</u>, 49–50
    processing of, 48
Williams, Serena, xviii
Williams, Venus, xviii, 23, 41
Woods, Tiger, 34

Workout partner. *See* Training partner
Wraps
    Guacamole Wraps, 121

Y

Yogurt
    Berry Parfait, 135
    Herbed Yogurt Cheese, 125
    Smoothie Pops, 128
Your Personal Health and Fitness Inventory, 9,
    <u>10–11</u>

Z

Zucchini
    Vegetable Frittata, 144